NTA UGC NET

Full Length Mock Test – Paper 2
Management
700 Practice Questions
with Explanations

(According to NTA UGC Latest Format)

Useful for:

NET/SET/SLET/PhD ENTRANCE/MANAGEMENT ENTRANCE EXAMS (ACROSS INDIA)

June 2025 Onwards

Dr. Ashima Negi

(PhD (Accounts), CA(I), MBA-Finance, PGDM-Supply Chain, BBA)
Guru Gobind Singh Indraprastha University
STATE GOVERNMENT UNIVERSITY
Government of NCT of Delhi, Delhi

Peepee Publishers and Distributors Private Limited®

NTA UGC NET Full Lenght Mock Test - Paper 2 Management
Author and Editor: Dr. Ashima Negix

Published by:
Pawaninder P. Vij and Anupam Vij

Peepee Publishers and Distributors Private Limited
Head Office: **160, Shakti Vihar, Pitam Pura, Delhi-110 034**

Correspondence Address:
7/31, First Floor, Ansari Road, Daryaganj
New Delhi-110002 (India)
Ph: 41512412, 9811156083
e-mail: **peepee160@yahoo.co.in**
e-mail: **peepee160@gmail.com**
www.peepeepub.com

First Edition: 2025

ISBN: 978-81-9833-660-6

Preface

Unlock your potential with "NTA UGC NET Management. Full length Mock Test with Solutions and crisp Explanations."

This essential element of your UGC NET Journey, offers a comprehensive collection of easy, complex and difficult full length mock tests and answer key, meticulously curated, provide in-depth and insightful explanations.

Perfect for aspirants aiming to master the **NTA UGC NET Management** exam.

This resource not only sharpens your problem-solving skills but also deepens your understanding of key concepts, through the explanations of question-answers. Equip yourself for success and navigate your path to achieving your academic career goals with confidence.

Preparing for the **NTA UGC NET Management** exam is a daunting task, but leveraging your practice with full length mock tests can significantly enhance your study strategy.

These tests are not only according to the latest exam pattern and question types but also serve as a valuable resource for self-assessment.

Are you feeling overwhelmed by the thought of preparing for the NTA UGC NET exam? You're not alone. Many aspirants find themselves wondering about the most effective way to tackle this challenging test AND only a few make it. This is your secret weapon to success.

The book is curated with Paper to help you against time element. By analysing past question's, I have identified key topics and areas which require focused study, to help you make you preparation more effective and efficient.

Through this book, I have delved into the significance of using mock tests by the students, for their preparation in **NTA UGC NET Management** exam.

Whether you are a first-time test-taker or looking to improve your score, this book aims to equip you with the tools needed for success, understanding how to leverage this book as a valuable resource can be a game-changer in your preparation journey.

Think of Management Mock Tests as your personal roadmap to exam success. This book offers you:

- A clear picture of the exam paper pattern
- Real examples of question types you'll face
- An effective tool for self-assessment
- Meticulously drafted topics and concepts

You will discover how to transform this resource into powerful tool for your exam success.

Let's revolutionize your preparation strategy !

Let's dive in and unlock the full potential in you. Because remember ..

"Success in the NET exam isn't just about studying harder—it's about studying smarter."

Dedication

Thank You Avani – Chiraag
Thank You Ba your Ashirwad always.*!!!*

MORE FROM THE HOUSE

- **Study Material -** According to the latest syllabus- Management.
- **Practice Manual –** With Unit wise 1000+ multi-choice questions.
- **Mock test(s)–** 7 Tests with 700+ practice questions, on all units of Management.
- **Previous Year Papers (Management) -**5 years- 9 Attempts, (Jan.2025 paper included).
- **Study Material** - According to the latest syllabus- Paper 1.
- **Practice Manual –** With Unit wise 1000+ multi-choice questions.
- **Mock test(s)** – 7 Tests including 700+ practice questions, covering all units of Paper 1.
- **Previous Year Papers (Paper 1) -** 5 years- 9 Attempts, (Jan.2025 paper included).
- **Dictionary (Research Aptitude) -**UGC NET, PhD, Research Professionals.

USP - List of MOST REPEATED TOPICs in NTA UGC NET.

- TOPICs wise list covered in every attempt in past 5 years exams in NTA UGC NET.

For more follow on –

Telegram – studytalkwithashima

Linkedin - www.linkedin.com/in/ashima-negi

Facebook - https://www.facebook.com/ashima.negi.3/

Academia - https://ggsipu.academia.edu/DrAshimaNegi

Contents

S.No.		*Page No.*
1	Practice Mock Test	1
2	Practice Mock Test	14
3	Practice Mock Test	28
4	Practice Mock Test	43
5	Practice Mock Test	57
6	Practice Mock Test	71
7	Practice Mock Test	84

UNIVERSITY GRANTS COMMISSION NET BUREAU

NET SYLLABUS

Subject : Management **Code No. 17**

Unit – I

- Management – Concept, Process, Theories and Approaches, Management Roles and Skills
- Functions – Planning, Organizing, Staffing, Coordinating and Controlling. Communication – Types, Process and Barriers.
- Decision Making – Concept, Process, Techniques and Tools
- Organisation Structure and Design – Types, Authority, Responsibility, Centralisation, Decentralisation and Span of Control
- Managerial Economics – Concept & Importance
- Demand analysis – Utility Analysis, Indifference Curve, Elasticity & Forecasting
- Market Structures – Market Classification & Price Determination
- National Income – Concept, Types and Measurement Inflation – Concept, Types and Measurement Business Ethics & CSR
- Ethical Issues & Dilemma Corporate Governance Value Based Organisation

Unit – II

- Organisational Behaviour – Significance & Theories
- Individual Behaviour – Personality, Perception, Values, Attitude, Learning and
- Motivation
- Group Behaviour – Team Building, Leadership, Group Dynamics
- Interpersonal Behaviour & Transactional Analysis
- Organizational Culture & Climate
- Work Force Diversity & Cross Culture Organisational Behaviour
- Emotions and Stress Management
- Organisational Justice and Whistle Blowing
- Human Resource Management – Concept, Perspectives, Influences and
- Recent Trends
- Human Resource Planning, Recruitment and Selection, Induction, Training and Development
- Job Analysis, Job Evaluation and Compensation Management

Unit – III

- Strategic Role of Human Resource Management Competency Mapping & Balanced Scoreboard Career Planning and Development
- Performance Management and Appraisal
- Organization Development, Change & OD Interventions
- Talent Management & Skill Development
- Employee Engagement & Work Life Balance
- Industrial Relations: Disputes & Grievance Management, Labour Welfare and
- Social Security
- Trade Union & Collective Bargaining
- International Human Resource Management – HR Challenge of International
- Business
- Green HRM

Unit– IV

- Accounting Principles and Standards, Preparation of Financial Statements
- Financial Statement Analysis – Ratio Analysis, Funds Flow and Cash Flow
- Analysis, DuPont Analysis
- Preparation of Cost Sheet, Marginal Costing, Cost Volume Profit Analysis
- Standard Costing & Variance Analysis
- Financial Management, Concept & Functions
- Capital Structure – Theories, Cost of Capital, Sources and Finance
- Budgeting and Budgetary Control, Types and Process, Zero base Budgeting
- Leverages – Operating, Financial and Combined Leverages, EBIT–EPS Analysis, Financial Breakeven Point & Indifference Level.

Unit –V

- Value & Returns – Time Preference for Money, Valuation of Bonds and Shares, Risk and Returns;
- Capital Budgeting – Nature of Investment, Evaluation, Comparison of Methods; Risk and Uncertainly Analysis
- Dividend – Theories and Determination
- Mergers and Acquisition – Corporate Restructuring, Value Creation, Merger
- Negotiations, Leveraged Buyouts, Takeover
- Portfolio Management – CAPM, APT
- Derivatives – Options, Option Payoffs, Option Pricing, Forward Contracts & Future Contracts
- Working Capital Management – Determinants, Cash, Inventory, Receivables and
- Payables Management, Factoring
- International Financial Management, Foreign exchange market

Unit - VI

- Strategic Management – Concept, Process, Decision & Types
- Strategic Analysis – External Analysis, PEST, Porter's Approach to industry analysis, Internal Analysis – Resource Based Approach, Value Chain Analysis
- Strategy Formulation – SWOT Analysis, Corporate Strategy – Growth, Stability, Retrenchment, Integration and Diversification, Business Portfolio Analysis - BCG, GE Business Model, Ansoff's Product Market Growth Matrix
- Strategy Implementation – Challenges of Change, Developing Programs
- Mckinsey 7s Framework
- Marketing – Concept, Orientation, Trends and Tasks, Customer Value and
- Satisfaction
- Market Segmentation, Positioning and Targeting
- Product and Pricing Decision – Product Mix, Product Life Cycle, New Product development, Pricing – Types and Strategies
- Place and promotion decision – Marketing channels and value networks, VMS, IMC, Advertising and Sales promotion

Unit –VII

- Consumer and Industrial Buying Behaviour: Theories and Models of Consumer
- Behaviour
- Brand Management – Role of Brands, Brand Equity, Equity Models, Developing a Branding Strategy; Brand Name Decisions, Brand Extensions and Loyalty
- Logistics and Supply Chain Management, Drivers, Value creation, Supply Chain
- Design, Designing and Managing Sales Force, Personal Selling
- Service Marketing – Managing Service Quality and Brands, Marketing Strategies of Service Firms
- Customer Relationship Marketing – Relationship Building, Strategies, Values and
- Process
- Retail Marketing – Recent Trends in India, Types of Retail Outlets.
- Emerging Trends in Marketing – Concept of e-Marketing, Direct Marketing, Digital Marketing and Green Marketing
- International Marketing – Entry Mode Decisions, Planning Marketing Mix for
- International Markets

Unit –VIII

- Statistics for Management: Concept, Measures Of Central Tendency and
- Dispersion, Probability Distribution – Binominal, Poison, Normal and Exponential
- Data Collection & Questionnaire Design
- Sampling – Concept, Process and Techniques
- Hypothesis Testing – Procedure; T, Z, F, Chi-square tests
- Correlation and Regression Analysis

- Operations Management – Role and Scope
- Facility Location and Layout – Site Selection and Analysis, Layout – Design and
- Process
- Enterprise Resource Planning – ERP Modules, ERP implementation
- Scheduling; Loading, Sequencing and Monitoring
- Quality Management and Statistical Quality Control, Quality Circles, Total Quality
- Management – KAIZEN, Benchmarking, Six Sigma; ISO 9000 Series Standards
- Operation Research – Transportation, Queuing Decision Theory, PERT / CPM

Unit –IX

- International Business – Managing Business in Globalization Era; Theories of
- International Trade; Balance of payment
- Foreign Direct Investment – Benefits and Costs
- Multilateral regulation of Trade and Investment under WTO International Trade Procedures and Documentation; EXIM Policies Role of International Financial Institutions – IMF and World Bank
- Information Technology – Use of Computers in Management Applications; MIS, DSS
- Artificial Intelligence and Big Data
- Data Warehousing, Data Mining and Knowledge Management – Concepts
- Managing Technological Change

Unit – X

- Entrepreneurship Development – Concept, Types, Theories and Process, Developing Entrepreneurial Competencies
- Intrapreneurship – Concept and Process
- Women Entrepreneurship and Rural Entrepreneurship
- Innovations in Business – Types of Innovations, Creating and Identifying
- Opportunities, Screening of Business Ideas
- Business Plan and Feasibility Analysis – Concept and Process of Technical, Market and Financial Analysis
- Micro and Small Scale Industries in India; Role of Government in Promoting SSI Sickness in Small Industries – Reasons and Rehabilitation
- Institutional Finance to Small Industries – Financial Institutions, Commercial
- Banks, Cooperative Banks, Micro Finance.

Practice Mock Test - 1

1) **Which of the following is necessary to understand banking rates of interest?**

a) Financial Statement Analysis

b) Capital Budgeting

c) Time Value of Money

d) All of the above

2) **Which app was opened as Atmanirbhar app, as an alternative to Twitter but was shut in July 2024?**

a) Chatter app

b) Chitter-Chatter app

c) Koo App

d) None of the above

3) **A store advertises a product at a low price but doesn't intend to sell it, instead convincing customers to buy a more expensive model.**

a) Insufficient stock

b) Bait and Switch

c) False Claims

d) Deceptive Advertising

4) **Which of the following is the goal of HR towards their efficient employees?**

a) Personnel workshop

b) Career Management

c) Career Plateau

d) All of the above

5) **Making promises of promotion but never following through. Displaying a lack of interest in the employee's career progress is known as**

a) Wallowing

b) Breadcrumbing

c) Ghosting

d) All of the above

6) **Which of the following sells the product at maximum retail price?**

a) Hyperstores

b) Dark stores

c) Mom and Pop Stores

d) All of the above

7) **Which of the following can be supported by a Natural Hazard Mitigation System?**

a) Floods

b) Tsunami

c) Earthquakes

d) All of the above

8) **A feeling of workplace disengagement resulting into a type of leave from employer is known as**

a) Casual Leave

b) Sick Leave

c) Mental Illness Leave

d) Unhappy Leave

9) **Which act covers welfare measures for working women?**

a) Maternity Benefits Act

b) Companies Act

c) Gratuity act

d) Factories Act

10) Which of the following concepts, essentially carry the Fundamental of Value Creation?

a) Product Concept

b) Selling Concept

c) Marketing Concept

d) Societal Marketing Concept

11) A store used by online Apps to hold and then disburse customer orders:

a) Hyperstore

b) Dark store

c) E-stores

d) E Commerce stores

12) Which committee/commission report is followed by NAAC, to implement Binary Accreditation System from Sept. 2024 onwards?

a) NEP 1968

b) NEP 2020

c) Radhakrishnan Committee

d) Acharya Ramamurti Committee.

13) Price gouging leads to stagflation, after demand shock period is over. True

14) If there is partial employment in the country, and competitive exams are negative processes of selection, educational qualification is a yardstick to earn livelihood, which is?

a) Economics of Development

b) Economics of Application

c) Economics of Discrimination

d) Both A and B

15) When aggregate income increases, consumption expenditure also increases but

a) By a somewhat large amount.

b) By a somewhat small amount.

c) Both A and B

d) None of the above.

16) A sample of 400 male students is found to have a mean height of 67.47 inches. Can it be regarded as a sample from a large population with mean height 67.39 inches and standard deviation. T

17) Bank submissions for overnight, 1/3/6/12 month <u>USD</u> settings will cease as of end June 2023 after which representative <u>LIBOR</u> rates will no longer be available.

a) USD

b) USD, LIBOR

c) INR

d) LIBOR

18) Which tradition after Ved- Anta, is part of spiritual discipline, according to Hindu Sadhana

a) Sankhya/Samkhya

b) Advait

c) Dvaita

d) Both A and C

19) A firm in late growth phase, decides on unrelated diversification from current product line. It's future call derivative will be signed at

a) Exercise price more than strike price.

b) Exercise price less than strike price.

c) Exercise price same as strike price.

d) None of the above

20) A performance appraisal technique that makes use of feedback rom supervisors, subordinates and co workers is known as :

a) Work oriented appraisal

b) 360 degree feedback

c) Informal appraisal

d) Graphic rating

21) **According to Hertzberg 2 Factor theory, which factors are not motivational factors?**

a) Satisfaction
b) Hygiene factors
c) Salary
d) None of the above

22) **Truck covers distance of 280 kms, speed is 40 kms/hour then time taken is 7 hours.**

23) **Research conducted in a new discipline is called**

a) Applied
b) Pure
c) Action
d) None of the above

24) **All apples are green. What is the symbol representing ?**

a) A
b) I
c) O

25) **Match the following:**

	LIST-I		LIST-II
A.	Web 1.0	I.	as a web of integration
B.	Web 2.0	II.	as a web of affiliation of websites
C.	Web 3.0	III.	Web of verbalization
D.	Web 4.0	IV.	Web of Static Information
E.	Web 5.0	V.	as a web of Decentralized Smart communication.

1. A-IV, B-III, C-II, D-I, E-V.
2. A-V, B-III, C-II, D-I, E-IV.
3. A-IV, B-V, C-II, D-I, E-III.
4. A-IV, B-V, C-I, D-II, E-III.

26) **_____ is a sequence of random words, stores data to access crypto-currency on blockchains/crypto wallets. Cryptocurrency wallets provide software that create _____**

a) D App, Seed Phrase
b) Seed Phrase, D App
c) Seed Phrase, Seed Phrase
d) D App, Web 3.0.

27) **Which applications can be built through a layer 1 protocol like 'Lisk'?**

a) Web 2.0 applications
b) Web 3.0 applications
c) Web 1.0 applications
d) Both A and C

28) **____ is a contract / financial instrument for an organization through which an employee when receives salary is supposed to payback a fixed % of their income.**

a) Compensation package
b) CTC
c) International Solar Alliance
d) Income Sharing Agreement

29) **According to which doctrine axing the law, if in case, some particular provision of a statute offends or is against a constitutional limitation, but that provision is severable from the rest of the statute, only that offending**

a) Doctrine severability
b) Doctrine of eclipse
c) Doctrine of waiver
d) Doctrine of territorial news

30) **____ contains a lost of central and state laws that cannot be challenged in court of law and was added by the constitution as the 1st amendment act, 1951, by the Govt of Pandit Nehru**

a) Schedule 12
b) Schedule 11
c) Schedule 9
d) Schedule 1

31) For economic growth and meeting the demands of inflation, the RBI Act 1934 recommended constitution of a statutory body as per

a) 4B(3C), RBI Act,1857

b) 45ZB, RBI Act, 1934

c) 45ZB, Constitutional Amendment Act, 1943

d) 54ZB, RBI Act,1938

32) Statement 1: Managers must develop healthy relations with various groups in order to achieve the goals smoothly.

Statement 2: Managers work only with internal people (subordinates, supervisors, peers) and not with external people.

a) Both 1 and 2 are correct

b) Both 1 and 2 are incorrect

c) Statement 1 is correct and statement 2 is incorrect

d) Statement 1 is incorrect and statement 2 is correct

33) An effective manager should make sure not to possess certain skills in the areas of planning, organizing, leading, controlling and decision making in order to process activities that are presented to him from time to time

a) Both Statement I and Statement II are correct.

b) Both statement I and Statement II are incorrect.

c) Statement I is correct and statement II is incorrect.

d) Statement I is incorrect and statement II is correct.

34) Statement 1: Managers play the figurehead role when they perform duties that are ceremonial and symbolic in nature.

Statement 2: Receiving and communicating information are perhaps the most important aspects of a manager.

a) Both 1 and 2 are correct

b) Both 1 and 2 are incorrect

c) Statement 1 is correct and statement 2 is incorrect

d) Statement 1 is incorrect and statement 2 is correct

35) Statement 1: An accounting manager supervises the accounting function

Statement 2: The manager of production supervises engineers and support staff engaged in design of a product or service.

a) Both 1 and 2 are correct

b) Both 1 and 2 are incorrect

c) Statement 1 is correct and statement 2 is incorrect

d) Statement 1 is incorrect and statement 2 is correct

36) Data cleaning is

a) Large collection of data mostly stored in a computer system.

b) Removal of noise errors and incorrect input from the database.

c) Systematic description of the syntactic structure of a specific database

d) None of these

37) Data scrubbing is

a) Process to reject data from the warehouse and to create the necessary indexes.

b) Process to load data into the warehouse and to create the necessary indexes.

c) A process to upgrade the quality of data after it is moved into the data warehouse.

d) A process to upgrade the quality of data before it is moved into the data warehouse.

38) ---- is held in the catalogue of the warehouse database system.

a) Application-level metadata.

b) Algorithm level metadata

c) Departmental level metadata

d) Core warehouse level metadata.

39) Among which of the following are NOT traditional theories in International Business

a) Porters five-forces theory

b) Comparative advantage theory

c) Hecker-Ohlin theory

d) Theory of Mercantilism

40) In web-mining --- is used to find natural groupings of mobiles, pagers.

a) Clustering

b) Associations

c) Sequential analysis

d) Classification

41) Which are the data mining tasks?

a) Regression

b) Classification

c) Clustering

d) All of the above

42) ----- maps the core warehouse metadata to business concepts, familiar and useful to end user.

a) Application-level metadata.

b) User level metadata.

c) End user level metadata.

d) Core level metadata

43) Which of the following related to CSR theories is correct?

a) Institutional theory is based on the shareholder concept

b) Social contract is the key concept of legitimacy theory.

c) Key concept of enlightened self-interest is stakeholder relations.

d) Stakeholder theory require organizations to manage community perceptions to survive.

44) Which of the following is correct related to discounting future liabilities?

a) Discounting future cash flows is not aligned with the aims and objectives of sustainability report.

b) Discounting future costs that are to be incurred increases the current liability.

c) Discounting future costs highlights the savings of the future generations due to present generations accounting.

d) Discounting social issues are done in terms of the accounting standards so that there are no ethical issues.

45) High commitment approach to environmental issues may include all of the following

a) Risk analysis

b) Stakeholder analysis

c) Green-washing

d) Strategic sustainability auditing

46) Which of the following statements regarding institutional shareholders is incorrect?

a) Have extensive power to monitor activities of the company.

b) Prefer to exert their power privately rather than publicly.

c) Aim to improve outcomes rather than sell their shareholding.

d) Institutional shares are known to publicly use their voting power to encourage sound corporate decision-making.

1. a, b, c.
2. b, c, d.
3. a, b, d.
4. All of the above.

47) Which of the following is not a driver of responsible competitiveness?

a) Policy drivers

b) Development drivers

c) Business action

d) Social enablers

48) The exit communication takes place when an employee ----- the organization

a) Enter into

b) Leaving from

c) Both

d) Leave

49) Audio visual communication is most suitable for mass publicity and mass *education.*

a) Publicity and education

b) Policies and political

c) Save and store

d) Educational policy

50) Unbounded solution in an LPP is

a) Where the objective function can be decreased indefinitely.

b) Which maximizes the objective function

c) Where the objective function can be increased or decreased indefinitely.

d) Where the objective function can be increased indefinitely.

51) The objective of the transportation problem is to

a) Maximize the total profit

b) Minimize the total loss

c) Neither maximize nor minimize

d) Optimal cost

52) If dark fruits chocolate was first priced by Amul at Rs 100, and then it was decreased by 5 % and later on increased by 7 %. The difference in the new and old price is

a) 102.45

b) 101.65

c) 2.34

d) 1.65

53) According to Sternberg there are 3 types of intelligence: Practical, creative and analytical T

54) Which market structure witness a demand kink, as the curve is more elastic above the kink and less elastic below it has because customer response to a price increase is less than the response to a price decrease.

a) Monopoly

b) Monopolistic competition

c) Oligopoly

d) Duopoly

55) Equilibrium is determined at the levels of output where

a) MC=MR

b) MC>MR

c) MC<MR

d) Both b and c

e) Both a and c

f) Both a and b

56) According to the managerial grid, which of the following management styles can be exercised by the organization.

1. a) Country club management, b) Team management, C) Improvised management, d) charismatic management
2. Country club management, b) Team management, c) Situational management. d) Task management

3. Country club management, b) Team management c) Impoverished, d) Task Management
4. None of the above.

57) Is the finite time and time that senior managers in a company possess. It is most often discussed when discussing the role and responsibilities of leaders and that many leaders take on more time than they can cry.

a) Administrative Theory
b) Scientific Management
c) Bandwidth Management
d) Management Bandwidth
e) Systems Management Theory

58) Customer decides not to join the queue by seeing the number of customers already in service system.

a) Balking
b) Reneging
c) Jockeying
d) Patient Customer

59) Customer after joining the queue, waits for some time and leaves the service due to delay in service.

a) Reneging
b) Jockeying
c) Balking
d) Impatient customer

60) If an activity has a total float of 10 minutes, with the latest start at 15th minute, then its earliest start is

a) 25 minutes
b) 10 minutes
c) 5 minutes
d) None of the above

61) If a project activity has pessimistic time of 9 minutes and optimistic time of 1 minute, with its most likely completion in 5 minutes. Then its variance is

a) 5 minutes
b) 2.56 minutes
c) 3.5 minutes
d) 9 minutes

62) A distribution which has equal tails, with a helping process of entire set of observations is called

a) Binomial distribution
b) Poisson Distribution
c) Beta Distribution
d) Normal Gaussian Distribution

63) A distribution of probability calculated by multiplying the probability of success raised to the power of the number of the successes and the probability of failure raised to the power of the difference between the number of is called

a) Poisson distribution
b) Gamma distribution
c) Cumulative Density Distribution
d) None of the above

64) Promotion of Zara Hatke Movie is

a) One to One marketing
b) Door to door selling
c) Road Show
d) Online promotion
e) Informative advertising

65) If Vicky Kaushal vibes on obsessed personalized only for you, this is called

a) Inter-personal communication
b) Extrinsic motivation
c) Attitude
d) Intrinsic motivation
e) Personality

66) According to you, which product is correctly combined with Market structure

a) Inferior goods- Perfect competition
b) Superior goods- Monopoly
c) Veblen goods - Monopolistic competition
d) Normal goods - oligopoly

67) Which of the following are modes of GAT's for supply of a service

a) Cross border
b) Consumption abroad
c) Commercial presence
d) All of the above
e) None of the above

68) Which of the following is not a vertical of World Bank Group?

a) IBRD
b) International Development Association (IDA)
c) General Agreement on Trade and Tariffs (GATTS)
d) The International Finance Corporation (IFC)
e) The Multilateral Investment Guarantee Agency

69) Identify incorrect formula

a) Sales-FC/EBIT
b) EBIT/EBT= Financial Leverage
c) Contribution - FC/EBIT-Interest = Financial Leverage
d) Contribution - FC/EBIT = Financial Leverage

70) Which theory states that "Consistency in judgement of people or issues linked by some form of relationship. Relationship of 3 elements- person, other person, impersonal entity, forming 2 relations- sentiment and unit (+ve, -ve)

a) Balance theory
b) Cognitive dissonance theory
c) Cognitive theory
d) None of the above
e) Alderfer ERG Theory

71) The following statement is true according to which theory: When cognitive components are incongruent, people will be motivated to alter their attitudes or behaviour to bring the whole back into balance.

a) Cognitive dissonance theory
b) Maslow's need hierarchy
c) ERG theory of motivation
d) Consistency theory of attitude

72) Identify the correct combination

a) MASLOW- ERG
b) PAC- Leadership Style
c) RoE- Accounting Concepts and Convention
d) NOI-Capital structure
e) None of the above

73) Which of the following is not an advantage of strategic management?

a) Provides organizations with a clear sense of direction and purpose.
b) Helps improve the political, economic, social and technological environment of the organization
c) Helps to orientate management decisions to relevant environment conditions
d) None of the above

74) Which of the following is not a characteristic of strategic management that makes it different from other type of management?

a) It is interdisciplinary
b) Has external focus
c) Has internal focus
d) Concerns present direction of the organization

75) The fundamental of a organization's mission statement is to

a) Create a good human relations climate in the organization

b) To define organization's purpose in society

c) Define organizational structure of the organization

d) Generate good public relations for the organization

76) If firm is at BEP, with FC of Rs.3 Lac and variable cost as 50 % of sales. Calculate units sold for selling price @ Rs 150/unit

a) 1500

b) 5000

c) 4000

d) 4900

e) 490

f) 1789

77) Receiving job satisfaction from your company is

a) Satisfier according to Herzberg 2-factor theory

b) Self Realization according to Maslow's need theory

c) Physiological need according to Maslow's need theory

d) None of the above

78) The board of directors work on behalf of stakeholders, this model is referred to as

a) Stakeholders model

b) Agency model

c) Ethical model

d) Anglo-Saxon model

79) If ABC Ltd issued 20% debentures for Rs 5 L and 1000 shares for Rs 15 L. EBIT is Rs 2 L Calculate D/E ratio and EAT if tax rate is 40%

a) 3:1, Rs 60,000

b) 2:1, Rs 1,00,000

c) 1:3, Rs 67,000

d) 1:3, Rs 40,000

e) 1:3, Rs 60,000

80) A leader calls in suggestions from his team members to improve customer satisfaction. Such style is called

a) Autocratic

b) Situational

c) Charismatic

d) None of the above

81) ____ is a RBI mandated system that offers integrated and interoperable bill payment services to customers across geographies to customers across geographies with certainty, reliability and safety of transactions.

a) UPI

b) Internet Banking

c) Mobile Banking

d) Bharat Bill Payment System

d) All of the above

e) None of the above

82) If an organization cleanliness is not maintained everyday, it will lead to extrinsic demotivation, leading to violation of which theory

a) Law of Demand

b) Law of Invariable Proportion

c) Maslow's need theory

d) Alderfer ERG theory

e) Herzberg's 2 factor theory.

83) If firm issues 20% dividend ratio for earnings per share of Rs 250, what is dividend paid?

a) Rs 25

b) Rs 65

c) Rs 50

d) None of the above

84) Which of the following explains that number of units of one product that can be increased by reducing the quantity of another product?

a) Marginal rate of substitution
b) Marginal rate of propensity
c) Marginal rate of transformation
d) All of the above

85) Which of the following explains that the amount of a good that a consumer is willing to consume as compared to another good, as long as the new good is equally satisfying:

a) Propensity to come
b) Demand function
c) Marginal rate of Substitution
d) Marginal rate of propensity

86) Which of the following is studied to evaluate how much quantity is to be produced by the firm?

a) Demand function
b) Cost function
c) Supply function
d) All of the above

87) Which body is responsible for printing/circulating Commemorative Coins in India

a) SEBI
b) UGC
c) RBI
d) SPMCIL (Security Printing and Minting Corporation of India Limited)

88) Which body is responsible for currency sterilization in India?

a) SEBI
b) Ministry of Corporate Affairs
c) UGC
d) AICTE
e) CABE
f) None of the above

89) If an investor sells below exercise price, on expiration date, then he will

a) Gain
b) Loose
c) No gain no loose
d) None of the above

90) Which ratio is useful if the firm wants to analyse the source of capital weightage?

a) Return on Investments Ratio
b) Return on Equity Ratio
c) Debt-Equity Ratio
d) Current Assets-Current Liabilities Ratio

91) A marketing analysis to improve return on investment, when the sales and marketing teams work together -

a) Word of mouth marketing
b) Digital marketing
c) Closed loop marketing
d) Both A and B

92) Ravi pointed to a girl in a picture, saying she is the mother of his child's grand-mother. How is Ravi related to the girl in the picture?

a) Son
b) Son In Law
c) Great Grand Mother
d) Great Grand Son

93) Which of the following can be checked by a potential investor before investing in an organization:

a) Balance sheet
b) Income/P&L statement
c) EBIT-EPS Analysis
d) Net Operating Income
e) Dividend Payout Ratio

94) RBI's clean note policy was introduced in

a) 2019, RBI Governor Dr Ustad Amjad Ali Khan
b) 1999, RBI Governor, Dr. Bimal Jain
c) 2001, RBI Governor, Dr. Nirmala S
d) 2007, RBI Governor, Dr. Radhe Shyam Tiwari

95) OD process is cyclical and ends when
a) Desired development result is obtained.
b) Plan is implemented
c) Data is gathered
d) Problem is identified

96) The organizational diagnosis means
a) To identify strength and weaknesses problem areas
b) To find out discrepancies, between vision and desired future and current situations
c) Both A and B
d) None of the above

97) OD was founded on the belief that using behavioural sciences methods to increase collaborative problem solving would increase
a) Organizational effectiveness
b) Organizational turnover
c) Organizational reputation
d) All of the above

98) OD Intervention seminars being conducted in the organisations help to
a) Improve overall efficiency
b) Improve productivity
c) Improve morale of employees
d) All the above

99) Which of the following is a performance management technique:
a) Essays
b) Write-ups
c) Observations
d) All of the above
e) None of the above

100)Which of the following is necessary for entrepreneurs to prepare when applying for venture capital or seeking seed funding
a) Business Report
b) Annual Financial Report
c) Feasibility analysis and Business Plan
d) None of the above

Answer Key Mock Test - 1

1 c) Time Value of Money
2 c) Koo App
3 b) Bait and Switch
4 b) Career Management
5 b) Breadcrumbing
6 c) Mom and Pop Stores
7 d) All of the above
8 d) Unhappy Leave
9 a) Maternity Benefits Act
10 c) Marketing Concept
11 d) E Commerce stores
12 c) Radhakrishnan Committee
13 TRUE
14 c) Economics of Discrimination
15 b) By a somewhat small amount.
16 TRUE
17 b) USD, LIBOR
18 b) Advait
19 b) Exercise price less than strike price.
20 b) 360 degree feedback
21 d) None of the above
22 distance covered 280 kms, speed is 40 kms/hour time taken is 7 hours.
23 b) Pure
24 a) A (Universal Affirmative)
25 1) A-IV, B-III, C-II, D-I, E-V.
26 c) Seed Phrase, Seed Phrase.
27 b) Web 3.0 applications
28 d) Income Sharing Agreement
29 a) Doctrine severability
30 c) Schedule 9
31 b) 45ZB, RBI Act, 1934
32 c) Statement 1 is correct and statement 2 is incorrect
33 d) Statement I is incorrect and statement II is correct.
34 a) Both 1 and 2 are correct
35 a) Both 1 and 2 are correct
36 b) Removal of noise errors and incorrect input from the database.
37 d) Upgrade the quality of data before moving to warehouse.
38 b) Algorithm level metadata
39 a) Porters five-forces theory
40 a) Clustering
41 d) All of the above
42 a) Application-level metadata.
43 b) Social contract is the key concept of legitimacy theory.
44 a) Discounting future cash flows not aligned to sustainability report.
45 c) Green-washing
46 1. a, b, c.
47 b) development drivers
48 b) Leaving from
49 a) Publicity and education
50 c) Where objective function is increased or decreased indefinitely.
51 a) Maximize the total profit
52 d) 1.65
53 True.
54 b) Monopolistic competition
55 e) Both a and c
56 3) Country club, b) Team, c) Impoverished, d) Task Management
57 d) Management Bandwidth
58 a) Balking
59 a) Reneging
60 c) 5 minutes
61 b) 5 minutes
62 d) Normal Gaussian Distribution
63 d) None of the above
64 e) Informative advertising
65 b) Extrinsic motivation
66 c) Veblen goods - Monopolistic competition
67 d) All of the above
68 c) General Agreement on Trade and Tariffs (GATTS)
69 a) Sales-FC/EBIT
70 a) Balance theory
71 a) Cognitive dissonance theory
72 d) NOI-Capital structure

73 d) None of the above
74 d) Concerns present direction of the organization
75 b) To define organization's purpose in society
76 c) 4000
77 a) Satisfier according to Herzberg 2-factor theory
78 b) Agency model
79 e) 1:3, Rs 60,000
80 d) None of the above
81 d) Bharat Bill Payment System
82 e) Herzberg's 2 factor theory.
83 c) Rs 50
84 c) Marginal rate of transformation
85 c) Marginal rate of Substitution
86 c) Supply function
87 d) SPMCIL (Security Printing & Minting Corporation of India)
88 f) None of the above
89 b) Loose
90 c) Debt-Equity Ratio
91 c) Closed loop marketing
92 d) Great Grand Son
93 c) EBIT-EPS Analysis
94 b) 1999, RBI Governor, Dr. Bimal Jain
95 a) Desired development result is obtained.
96 c) Both A and B
97 a) Organizational effectiveness
98 d) All the above
99 c) Observations
100 c) Feasibility analysis and Business Plan

Practice Mock Test - 2

101) **STATEMENT I - Action research is for finding answer to immediate problems at hand.**

STATEMENT II - Applied research is the same as action research, both involve interviewing the respondents.

a) Both STATEMENT I and STATEMENT II are correct.

b) Both STATEMENT I and STATEMENT II are incorrect.

c) STATEMENT I is correct and STATEMENT II is incorrect.

d) STATEMENT I is incorrect and STATEMENT II is correct.

102) **STATEMENT I - Pure researched that generate data for the first time, in a field, where no research was done, ever.**

STATEMENT II - Fundamental researches help add data to existing subject knowledge.

a) Both STATEMENT I and STATEMENT II are correct.

b) Both STATEMENT I and STATEMENT II are incorrect.

c) STATEMENT I is correct and STATEMENT II is incorrect.

d) STATEMENT I is incorrect and STATEMENT II is correct.

103) **STATEMENT I - Any research requires primary data to support its hypothesis.**

STATEMENT II - Research type is based on the format of research reporting, as well.

a) Both STATEMENT I and STATEMENT II are correct.

b) Both STATEMENT I and STATEMENT II are incorrect.

c) STATEMENT I is correct and STATEMENT II is incorrect.

d) STATEMENT I is incorrect and STATEMENT II is correct.

104) **STATEMENT I - Most important element in research is termed as research analysis, only.**

STATEMENT II - Research hypothesis is always self-explanatory in itself.

a) Both STATEMENT I and STATEMENT II are correct.

b) Both STATEMENT I and STATEMENT II are incorrect.

c) STATEMENT I is correct and STATEMENT II is incorrect.

d) STATEMENT I is incorrect and STATEMENT II is correct.

105) **STATEMENT I - All types of Research end up using same design of research.**

STATEMENT II - All research types conduct data analysis.

a) Both STATEMENT I and STATEMENT II are correct.

b) Both STATEMENT I and STATEMENT II are incorrect.

c) STATEMENT I is correct and STATEMENT II is incorrect.

d) STATEMENT I is incorrect and STATEMENT II is correct.

106) STATEMENT I - Most important element of sampling stage is to prepare sampling frame.

STATEMENT II - Most important element in reporting is to give references & citations and data analysis.

a) Both STATEMENT I and STATEMENT II are correct.

b) Both STATEMENT I and STATEMENT II are incorrect.

c) STATEMENT I is correct and STATEMENT II is incorrect.

d) STATEMENT I is incorrect and STATEMENT II is correct.

107) STATEMENT I - Research Design carries types of research methods to be used for the research.

STATEMENT II - Data Analysis Technique Chi Square Method is conducted in quantitative data, only.

a) Both STATEMENT I and STATEMENT II are correct.

b) Both STATEMENT I and STATEMENT II are incorrect.

c) STATEMENT I is correct and STATEMENT II is incorrect.

d) STATEMENT I is incorrect and STATEMENT II is correct.

108) STATEMENT I - Primary data collection is possible through survey method.

STATEMENT II - Research synopsis is prepared like the research proposal, in same fashion.

a) Both STATEMENT I and STATEMENT II are correct.

b) Both STATEMENT I and STATEMENT II are incorrect.

c) STATEMENT I is correct and STATEMENT II is incorrect.

d) STATEMENT I is incorrect and STATEMENT II is correct.

109) STATEMENT I - Research hypothesis can be based on pilot study findings.

STATEMENT II - Research hypothesis formulation mandatory to involve literature review.

a) Both STATEMENT I and STATEMENT II are correct.

b) Both STATEMENT I and STATEMENT II are incorrect.

c) STATEMENT I is correct and STATEMENT II is incorrect.

d) STATEMENT I is incorrect and STATEMENT II is correct.

110) STATEMENT I - Research article is presented in seminars and colloquiums.

STATEMENT II - White papers do not involve extensive researches.

a) Both STATEMENT I and STATEMENT II are correct.

b) Both STATEMENT I and STATEMENT II are incorrect.

c) STATEMENT I is correct and STATEMENT II is incorrect.

d) STATEMENT I is incorrect and STATEMENT II is correct.

111) Which of the following discipline discusses need for understanding the organization's climate for better improvement towards employee coordination?

a) Principles of Management

b) Practices of Marketing

c) Organizational Behaviour

d) None of the above

112) Which of the following leadership styles can be used when leaders seek inputs from team members:

a) Situational leadership style.

b) Autocratic leadership style.

c) Participative leadership style.

d) All of the above

e) None of the above

113) Which of the following can be used for evaluation and taking investment decisions for financial management.

a) Time Value of Money

b) Net Present Value

c) Cost of Equity Debt

d) Security Market Line

114) A distributed 10% preferred dividend on Net Income of Rs 15 L and had a long term source of capital in form of equity shares of Rs 10. L

a) 1

b) 1.5

c) 1.35

d) 2.10

115) If sales is 5 L , variable cost is 40% of sales and fixed cost is 1 L. Then operating leverage is

a) 2.5

b) 3

c) 2.95

d) None of the above

116) Raja left for work and cycled 5 km south, he took a left turn and walked 2 km to office Which direction he ends his journey?

a) West

b) South west

c) South

d) East

e) North

117) Ram is being overburdened, as his boss Ravi a lot of work. Which Henry Fayol's principle is applied here:

a) E spirit De Corps

b) Principle of renumeration

c) Unity of direction

d) All of the above

e) None of the above

118) Ravi pointed to a picture and said, the boy in the picture is the son of my sister's husband. How is Ravi related to the boy in the picture.

a) Paternal Uncle

b) Paternal grandfather

c) Maternal uncle

d) Brother Cousin

119) Which of the following theory lays importance upon building harmonious relationships with the organization and the society

a) Herzberg 2 factor theory

b) Theory of emotional intelligence

c) Maslow's hierarchy needs theory

d) Hnery Fayol's 14 principles

120) Ram left for work at 8 am, cycling 8 km north, took a right turn and walked 3 km. Then he took another right to ride on a bike with an office colleague for 8 km. How far is he from starting point?

a) 19 km

b) 8 km

c) 3 km

d) 8.544 km

121) Which of the following is correct input to assess the organizational structure?

a) Attitudes, norms and salaries

b) Values, bonus and norms

c) Attitudes, Norms and Values

d) All of the above

122) Identify the regulatory body for quality standards in India (NTA)

a) RBI

b) AICTE

c) CABE

d) UGC

123) Which of the following is a finance function?

a) Distribution of dividends

b) Calculating leverages on operations

c) Issue of shares and debentures

d) All of the above

124) Identify the college which is in the top 3 NIRF Rankings 2022 and was opened by Britishers

a) Elphinstone Institution

b) All India Institute of Medical Sciences

c) IIM Ahmedabad

d) Presidency College

125) Which of the following bodies has the objective to restructure curriculum in India

a) CARE

b) MoE

c) UGC

d) NCTE

126) What is the aspect ratio of IMAX theatre where a movie Pathan was screened shot exclusively on IMAX cameras

a) 1.43: 1

b) 5.31: 1

c) 2.43:1

d) 1.43: 3

127) If a firm incurs cost of preference shares (kp) 15.65% carrying redemption value of Rs 3 L, for net proceeds of 2 L for 2 years lock in period. Then total preferred dividend paid is Rs 39125

a) Correct

b) Incorrect

128) If a firm pays dividend in 2019 and 2023 @5.65% DPR, when IRR is 15 %, cost of equity is 13.2 and EPS is Rs 128

a) Dividend of both years will be different.

b) Dividend of both years will be same

c) Both a and b

d) None of the above

129) What is proposition for Contrapositive form "Some non people are not non gripe"

a) All non-people are non-gripe

b) Some gripe are not people

c) Some people are not gripe

d) None of the above

130) If material cost variance is 5600 (adverse) and standard expenses for 1000 kg are Rs 10 per unit, then total actual expenses for 1500 kg are

a) Rs15

b) Rs 10

c) Rs 10.46

d) Rs 10.4

e) Rs 11.98

131) If Net Operating Income is Rs 10,000 and fixed cost is Rs 15,000 calculate variable cost which is 20% of sales revenue

a) 25,000

b) 6250

c) 31,250

d) 64,250

132) If EBIT is Rs 8 L and Pretax Income is 60% of EBIT. The equity invested by shareholders is Rs 10 L and 150 % of equity was invested by the organization in total assets. The firm generated Rs 3 L of net Income, when it's operating revenue is

a) Revenue = Rs 10 L, RoE=0.3015

b) Revenue = Rs 1 L, RoE=0.6

c) Revenue = Rs 15 L, RoE=0.72

d) None of the above

133) IF ABC Ltd has Tax Burden of 1.67 with net income of Rs 5 L , find out Pretax Profit

a) 13 L

b) 12 L

c) 5 L

d) 23 L

e) 3 L

134) With EBIT at 16 L and interest coverage ratio being 4 times, EAT is calculated to be 6 L. What is the tax paid?

a) 4 L

b) 6 L

c) 16 L

d) 12 L

e) None of the above

135) By how much % has the EPFO (Employee Provident Fund Organization) increased the interest rate for the financial year 2022-2023?

a) 8.15

b) 9

c) 8.5

d) 7.5

136) Which of the following is attended by learners to improve and increase industrial knowledge?

a) Capstone Project

b) Seminar

c) Colloquium

d) Conference

137) If std. expenses for manufacturing 100 units is Rs 12,000, consuming 1000 kg raw material. Today firm is planning to produce 200 units, using 1500 kg raw material for Rs 10/kg. The material cost variance is

a) Favourable

b) Adverse

c) Nil

138) What is it called when a client takes orders from the clients and then finds cheap free lancers to complete the client order

a) Order retailing

b) Drop servicing/service arbitrage/ white labelling

c) Free servicing

d) All of the above

139) Identify the missing series 3,8, 27, ___, 565

a) 56

b) 122

c) 112

d) 84

140) A test which has been recently banned by Supreme Court and the professional performing it shall be penalized

a) Chi square test

b) F Test

c) 2 finger test

d) Kruskal wallis test

141) According to which constitutional amendment, EWS based reservation NOT to be merged in 50% reservation.

a) 46th Constitutional Amendment, 1976

b) 103rd Constitutional Amendment, 2019

c) 23rd Constitutional Amendment, 2022

142) Landmark judgement (2022) to rehabilitate sex workers back into the society, through vocational skill-based training, by a three-judge bench was given in the case of

a) Budhadev Karmakar Vs State of West Bengal

b) Union of India vs Kejriwal Govt.

c) Union of India vs ND Modi

143) Research undertaken to find solutions for testing a theory on selected few sections of the population is called

a) Action Research

b) Applied Research

c) Inductive Research

d) Deductive Research

e) Exploratory Research

144) Which Hindu philosopher wrote Mimamsa philosophy of thought

a) Adi Shankaracharya

b) Mandan Mishra

c) Shankacharya Swaropanand Saraswati

d) None of the above

145) UN declares 2023 as

a) International Millets Year

b) International Water Conservation Year

c) International Forests Year

d) All of the above

146) CERT – in observes Cyber Jaagrooka Diwas on ... to create awareness and sensitize Internet Users on safeguarding against cyber frauds and cybercrimes.

a) 01st July

b) 01st August

c) 01st December

d) 01st November

e) 01st June

147) Reserve Bank will conduct open market purchase of government securities under the G-sec Acquisition programme (2.0) for an aggregate amount of Rs 15,000 crore on September 30,2021

a) Gsap-RBI

b) RBI Core solutions

c) Shares equity

d) Company deposits

148) Monetary policy strategy used by central banks aimed at stimulating economic growth through lowering long-term interest rates. This is achieved by selling near- term treasuries to buy longer dated ones

a) Strategic twist

b) Corporate Strategy

c) Operation Twist

d) Core Solutions

149) National Payments Corporation of India (NPCI), Department of Financial Services (DFS), National Health Authority (NHA), Ministry of Health and Family Welfare (MoHFW) and partner banks has launched an innovative digital solution.

a) UPI Gateway

b) BHIM UPI

c) What's App UPI

d) e-RUPI

150) Govt of India, Ministry of Finance, jointly with RBI has announced series I and Series II of Sovereign Gold Bond (SGB) 2022-23. Identify the portal on which the SGB shall be accessed by investors.

a) RBI.com

b) MOF.ac.in

c) GoI portal

d) e-kuber portal

151) Online platform used by Delhi University to reach its students online is

a) Google chrome

b) Google classes

c) Google hangouts.

d) Both B and C

152) India International Arbitration Centre3 was previously known as New Delhi International Arbitration Centre.

True

False

153) An Altman Z Score suggests that a company has financial distress and has greater chances of going bankrupt.

True

False

154) Correct Formula for Sloan Ratio

a) (NET INCOME-CFO-CFI) + Total Assets

b) (NET INCOME-CFO-CFI) X Fixed Assets

c) (NET INCOME-CFO-CFI) / Fixed Assets

d) (NET INCOME-CFO-CFI) / Total Assets

155) Researchers are unethical when

a) Collect data from respondents

b) Conducting disguised observations

c) All of the above

156) Identify incorrect pair

a) NPV - Investment decision

b) DPR-Dividends decision

c) BOE- Financing decision

d) All of the above

157) Positivistic research is

a) Qualitative research

b) Quantitative research

c) Empirical research

d) Inductive research

158) Vaccines are made from buffalo skin. This is a fallacy of

a) Appeal to pity.

b) Appeal to emotion

c) Appeal to tradition.

d) Appeal to nature

159) If response recorded from a respondent is incorrect researcher changes it by himself, it is a case of

a) Biasness

b) Unethical practices

160) 3rd July is

a) International Women's Day

b) International Men's Day

c) International Plastic Bag Free Day

d) International Ozone Day

161) Ram is being overburdened, as his boss Ravi and sita's boss Krishnan have given Ram a lot of work. Which Henry Fayol's Principle is applied here:

1) Esprit De Corps
2) Principle of Remuneration
3) Unity of Command
4) All of the Above
5) None of the Above

162) A is lively and carefree in his attitude. The temperament he has is known as

a) sanguine
b) melancholic
c) Choleric
d) Phlegmatic

163) Which of the following explains that number of units of one product that can be increased by reducing the quantity of another product.

1) Marginal rate of substitution
2) Marginal rate of propensity
3) Marginal rate of transformation

164) Which of the following leadership styles can be used when leaders do not wish to seek inputs from team members:

a) Participative Leadership Style
b) Autocratic Leadership Style
c) Democratic Leadership Style
d) Situational Leadership Style

165) Which of the following discipline discusses need for understanding the organisations climate for better improvement towards employee coordination

a) Organisational Development
b) Organisational Behaviour
c) Organisational Process
d) A and C

166) OD intervention seminars being conducted in the organizations help to:

1) Improve overall efficiency
2) Improve Productivity
3) Improve morale of the employee

167) A leader calls in suggestions from his team members to improve customer satisfaction. Such style is called

a) Participative Leadership Style
b) Autocratic Leadership Style
c) Democratic Leadership Style
d) Situational Leadership Style

168) The following statement is true according to which theory: "When cognitive components are incongruent, people will be motivated to alter their attitudes or behaviour to bring the whole back into balance".

a) Elaboration theory of Attitude
b) Social judgement theory of Attitude
c) Cognitive theory of dissonance
d) Consistency theory of Attitude

169) .... is an RBI mandated system which offers integrated and interoperable bill payment services to customers across geographies with certainty, reliability and safety of transactions.

1) UPI
2) Internet Banking
3) Mobile Banking
4) Bharat Bill Payment System

170) Identify the simulation models

a) Dynamic simulation

b) Static simulation

c) Discrete simulation

d) Continuous simulation

e) None of the above

f) All of the above

171) If standard costs are Rs 50,000, actual costs are Rs 36,000, then material cost variance is

a) Rs 14,000 adverse

b) Rs 14,000 favourable

c) Rs 36,000 adverse

d) Rs 50,000 favourable

172) Assertion: Loss % is calculated by reducing sales value minus cost price.

Reason: Speed is calculated by multiplying distance with time

a) Both ASSERTION and REASON are true and REASON is correct explanation

b) Both ASSERTION and REASON are true and REASON IS not the correct explanation

c) ASSERTION is true but REASON is false

d) ASSERTION is false but REASON is true.

173) Dividend Theories which help calculate the price of shares

a) MM theory

b) Dividend Irrelevancy Theory

c) Walter theory

d) Gordon theory

e) Dividend yield approach

1) A and B

2) C and D

3) D and E

4) A and E.

174) Carbon emission controlling protocols:

a) Rio Summit

b) Kyoto

c) Paris Accord

d) Millennium development goals

e) Sustainable development goals

1) A & B

2) B & C

3) A & C

4) C & E

175) If current ratio is -4.5:1. non-current liabilities: current liabilities is 2:1. And non -current liabilities are Rs 2 L. Calculate current assets

a) Rs 2 L

b) Rs 45,000

c) Rs 1,00,000

d) Rs 4,50,000

176) Equal likelihood criterion multiplies the decision payoff for each alternative solution by an equal weight, thus assuming that the alternatives are equally likely to occur. This criterion is also called

a) Hurwicz creation

b) Laplace Criterion

c) Both a and b

d) None of the above

177) We guarantee coverage for your project. Our criterions for eligibility include

a) Non-Honouring of financial obligations

b) Appropriation

c) War and Civil disturbance
d) Expropriation
e) Breach of contract
f) Currency inconvertibility
1. A, B, C, D.
2. A, C, D, E, F
3. B, C, D, E, F
4. A, C, D, F.

178) We provide political risk insurance and credit enhancement for cross border private sector investors and lenders. Who are we?

a) IMF
b) MSME
c) Khadi Commission
d) Multilateral Investment Guarantee Agency

179) If a respondent does not give full/ accurate information in the research questionnaire, this situation is called

a) Respondent bias
b) Questionnaire error
c) Sampling Error
d) Both a and c

180) Champions.gov.in website is for

a) Creation and Harmonious application of modern Processes for increasing Output and National Strength.
b) Credit and Harmonious application of modern Processes for increasing Output and National Strength.
c) Creation and Harmonious application of modern Processes for increasing Output and National Income.
d) Creation and Harmonious application of medium Processes for increasing Output and National Strength.

181) A KVIC portal for credit linked subsidy, where beneficiary gets 15-35% of total project cost from government

a) PM KVIC Scheme
b) PM Employment
c) PM Credit-linked Scheme
d) PMeGP

182) A platform keeping track of various procurements done from MSME Sector

a) MAME SAMBANDH
b) MSME UDYAM
c) MSME Act, 2006
d) Both b and c

183) A platform for free of cost registration for entrepreneurs and MSME for self- declaration is called

a) MSME Registration portal
b) MSME Act, 2006
c) MSME Udyam Portal
d) MSME KVIC Portal

184) Which world bank group body offers standby credit arrangement?

a) MIGA
b) IBRD
c) IMF
d) ICSID

185) PLC returns diminish if

a) Company is in introduction stage
b) Sales increase beyond average production
c) Sales reduce
d) Average production reduces
e) Marginal cost increases than marginal revenue

186) The strategy that chooses the alternative with highest average payoff is called

a) Expansion strategy

b) Laplace Strategy

c) Unrelated Diversification Strategy

d) Both A and C

187) If standard price and standard quantity are more than actual price and actual quantity then

a) There is a favourable variance

b) No variance

c) There is a adverse variance

d) None of the above

188) A retailer which has bulk storage and selling price is either discounted or is based on psychological prices:

a) Mom n Pop Store

b) Supermarkets

c) Both a and b

d) EDLP stores

e) Speciality stores

189) Variances are found in cases of

a) Risk

b) Costs

c) Profits

d) Both a and b

e) Both b and c

190) If risk free rate of return is 10 % and market-based returns are 15 % with systematic risk at 1.95, calculate CAPM

a) 19.75%

b) 18 %

c) 15 %

d) 11 %

191) If a firm has annual demand of cash for Rs 1,20,000 and fixed transaction cost it has to pay for is Rs 250 and opportunity cost is 8 %. Then EOQ of cash is

a) 25,000

b) 10000

c) 38276

d) 27386

192) Recently banned food item by India in 2022 is

a) Rice

b) Crude Oil

c) Petrol

d) Wheat

e) Oatmeal

193) Commerce and Management micro finance can be availed by

a) Corporate Ventureast

b) Big Business houses

c) Small business houses

d) Small scale individual entrepreneurs

e) Women entrepreneurs and rural entrepreneurs

194) What is more of a foundation to begin research from grass root level?

a) Research hypothesis

b) Research Methodology

c) Research question

d) Both a and b

195) Non uses of cash flow statement

a) Recording cash outflow and inflow

b) Helpful in cash management'

c) Helpful in financial management

d) All of the above

e) None of the above

196) Identify important features of Credit Policy of an organization

a) Credit period

b) Credit standards

c) Credit Appraisal

1) Both B and C

2) Both A and C

3) Both A and B

197) SUAVE: SOPHISTICATED

a) Attitude: conduct

b) Adage: language

c) Calmness: placidity

d) Ally: foe

198) Identify the missing letter/number from the given alternatives AFN, MQZ, CGP

a) OSB

b) PUE

c) MPX

d) OTC

199) If a response is not given to an emailed Google form questionnaire then following is committed

a) Respondent's bias

b) Non response error

c) Wrong Variable

d) Sampling error

200) Served from India scheme was replaced with

a) FTP: 2015-2020

b) FTP: 2021-2026

c) Service Exports from India Scheme

d) EXIM Policy

Answer Key Mock Test - 2

101 c)
102 c)
103 b)
104 b)
105 d)
106 a)
107 c)
108 c)
109 c)
110 c)
111 c) Organizational Behaviour
112 c) Participative leadership style.
113 b) Net Present Value
114 c) 1.35
115 d) None of the above
116 d) East
117 e) None of the above
118 c) Maternal uncle
119 c) Maslow's hierarchy needs theory
120 c) 3 km
121 d) All of the above
122 d) UGC
123 a) Distribution of dividends
124 d) Presidency College
125 c) UGC
126 a) 1.43: 1
127 a) Correct
128 b) Dividend of both years will be same
129 b) Some gripe are not people
130 d) Rs 10.4
131 b) 6250
132 a) Revenue = Rs 10 L, RoE=0.3015
133 e) 3 L
134 b) 6 L
135 a) 8.15
136 c) Colloquium
137 a) Favourable
138 b) Drop servicing/service arbitrage/ white labelling
139 c) 112
140 c) 2 finger test
141 b) 103rd Constitutional Amendment, 2019
142 a) Budhadev Karmakar Vs State of West Bengal
143 c) Inductive Research
144 b) Mandan Mishr
145 a) International Millets Year
146 e) 01st June
147 a) Gsap-RBI
148 c) Operation Twist
149 d) e-RUPI
150 d) e-kuber portal
151 d) Both B and C
152 TRUE
153 TRUE
154 d) (NET INCOME-CFO-CFI) / Total Assets
155 a) Collect data from respondents
156 c) BOE- Financing decision
157 c) Empirical research
158 d) Appeal to nature
159 b) Unethical practices
160 c) International Plastic Bag Free Day
161 None
162 Sanguine
163 Marginal rate of transformation
164 Autocratic Leadership Style
165 Organisational Behaviour
166 All of the Above
167 Participative Leadership Style
168 Consistency theory of Attitude
169 d) All of the Above
170 f) All of the above
171 b) Rs 14,000 favourable
172 d) ASSERTION is false but REASON is true.
173 3) D & E
174 2) B & C
175 d) Rs 4,50,000
176 b) Laplace Criterion
177 A, C, D, E, F
178 d) Multilateral Investment Guarantee Agency
179 a) Respondent bias
180 a) Creation and Harmonious application of modern Processes.
181 d) PMeGP

182 d) Both b and c
183 c) MSME Udyam Portal
184 c) IMF
185 d) Average production reduces
186 b) Laplace Strategy
187 a) There is a favourable variance
188 b) Supermarkets
189 d) Both a and b
190 a) 19.75%
191 c) 38276
192 d) Wheat
193 d) Small scale individual entrepreneurs
194 c) Research question
195 e) None of the above
196 3) Both A and B
197 c) Calmness: placidity
198 a) OSB
199 b) Non response error
200 c) Service Exports from India Scheme

Practice Mock Test - 3

201) Policy merged different schemes under Merchandise Export from India scheme" (MEIS) The different schemes were

a) Market Linked Focus Product Scheme

b) Infrastructure Incentive Scrip

c) Focus Market Scheme

d) Service Exports from India Scheme

202) Key focus of foreign trade policy 021-2026

a) To make India a 5 trillion S economy

b) To boost imports

c) To bring changes to regulatory and operational framework and lower the transactional costs of Foreign Trade Policy

d) Both A and B

e) Both A, C

f) All of the above

203) Which of the following is necessary to exist in the research?

a) Validity

b) Reliability

c) Objectivity

d) AOA

e) None

204) What is important in research?

a) Research Design

b) Sampling Technique

c) APA/MLA/Chicago Format

d) Research Process

205) Identify incorrect COVID vaccine

a) COVISHEILD

b) COVAXIN

c) Johnson and Johnson Vaccine

d) Moderna Vaccine

e) Sputnik V Vaccine

f) Zydus Cadilla Vaccine

g) Unnat Bharat Vaccine

206) Which are the 4 categories in SDG India Index Report 2021?

a) Aspirant-> Performer-> Front Runner-> Achiever

b) Aspirant-> Runner-> Performer-> Achiever

c) Front Runner ->Aspirant-> Performer-> Achiever

d) Achiever-> Performer-> Front Runner ->Aspirants

207) Top achiever as per the SDG India Report 2021

a) Kerela + Delhi

b) Karnataka + Daman

c) Karnataka + Chandigarh

d) Kerela + Chandigarh

208) Identify the correct combination

a) School Education – 100 %, 2025

b) Higher Education, 50%, 2035

c) School Education - 100%, 2030

d) Higher Education - 50 %, 2035

1. A and B

2. B and C

3. B and D

209) Foundation Literacy & Numeracy in NEP 2020 is for

a) School Education

b) Angadwadi

c) 10+2+3

d) 5+3+3+4

e) Higher Education

210) Curriculum updation is done by

a) Executive Council

b) Academic Council

c) UGC

d) College Director/HOD

211) HECI verticals focus on

a) Regulations+ Research+ Grants+ Accreditation

b) Regulations+ Education + Research+ Grants+ Accreditation

c) Research+ Grants+ Accreditation + Distance Education

d) Research + Distance Education + Accreditation + Grants

212) Light but tight for NEP 2020 stands for

a) Syllabus

b) Research

c) Regulations

d) All of the above

e) None of the above

213) Panini wrote which book?

a) Nyaya sutra

b) Yoganacare

c) Ashtadhyayi

d) Navaiddhi

214) NIRF 2021 Best College Rankings

a) IIT Madras> IISc Bengaluru> IIT Delhi

b) Miranda House> Lady Shri Ram College > Loyola College

c) IIT Madras< IISc Bengaluru< IIT Delhi

d) Delhi University> IISc Bengaluru> Mumbai University

215) India's 1st open University is

a) Indira Gandhi National Open University, 1985

b) Maharashi Dayanand University, 1976

c) IGNOU, 1986

d) Dr. B.R. Ambedkar Univesity, 1982

216) Management Investor gets dividend that's more than he expected, then he can re-invest in the company's stock with the surplus cash flow

a) MM's approach to dividend

b) Walter approach to dividend

c) Gordon approach to dividend

d) Irrelevancy approach to dividend

217) ______ is the theory of knowledge that deals with how knowledge is gathered and from which sources

a) Research Methodology

b) Pre- Research study

c) Research methods

d) Research Epistemology

218) Most authentic internal source of finance is

a) Shares + Debentures + Preferred Stock

b) Shares + Retained Earnings + Preferred Stock

c) Shares + Retained Earnings + Promoters Capital

d) Retained Earnings + Promoters Capital+ Deferred expenses

219) Most important for any entrepreneur is

a) Preparation of business plan

b) Getting loan Approval

c) Getting government approval of project

d) Getting good and dedicated staff

220) Which of the following combination is bad.

a) Coconut trees + Water bodies

b) Mines + Oil drilling sites

c) Agricultural fields + Water Bodies

d) Residential area + Nuclear plant

221) Teaching aids are useful for

a) While making colourful data presentations

b) While making understand deaf and mute learners

c) While creating a 1st impression on new batch.

d) While highlighting key points

222) Match the following

a) Research Paper	I) Experience discussion
b) Paper Presentation	II) Paper presentation
c) Conference	III) Article publication

Choose the correct answer:

a) A-II, B-III, C-I

b) A-II, B-III, C-I

c) A-III, B-II, C-I

223) Match the following

a) BCG Matrix	I) Industry Competitiveness
b) Ansoff Matrix	II. Market Share
c) Cell Matrix	III. Existing /New Markets

Choose the correct answer:

a) A-I, B-II, C-III

b) A-II, B-III, C-I

c) A-III, B-II, C-I

224) India by 2020 aims to create ______ to consume 2.5-3.0 Billion of CO2, creating additional forest cover.

a) Greenhouse gas

b) Solar panels

c) Carbon footprint

d) Carbon Sink

e) Carbon Emissions

225) India's INDC's commitment to reduce emission intensity by 2030 is

a) 3-5% of GDP

b) 33-35% of NDP

c) 75% of GDP

d) 33-35 % of GDP

226) Given by E, D. Wilson, this term means variability amongst living organisms and ecological diversities. It is called

a) Ecosystem

b) Biological and aquatic ecosystems

c) Biodiversity

d) Ecology

227) Mr. Chirag (a researcher, Thermo-dynamics) talks to Mr. Ram (a M.Tech student), who answered a few questions for Mr. Chirag. And further asked him to talk to Ms. Rosy (a Mechanical Engineer). This is

a) Research study

b) Obtaining informed consent

c) Snowball sampling

d) Data collection

228) Which of the following is incorrect pair?

a) Mimasa and Vedanta

b) Nyaya and Vaisheshika

c) Lokayara and Kapalika

d) Lokayata and Kapalika

229) a) Sankhya is not accepting rebirth of soul

b) Self - knowledge leads to liberation

Which statement is correct?

a) 1 only

b) 2 only

c) Both 1 and 2

d) Neither 1 or 2

230) P1: All the apples are in the basket

P2: Few Apples are rotten

Conclusion: Some apples maybe are ripe

a) Inductive argument

b) Deductive argument

c) Inductive valid argument

d) Deductive valid argument

231) If "No Apricots are real" is taken to be true, then false proposition is

a) Some apricots are big.

b) All apricots are big.

c) Some apricots are real

d) Some apricots are not big

e) Some apricots are there

232) Highest educational advisory body in India who advises to state and central government

a) UGC

b) NTA

c) AICTE

d) CABE

e) Ministry of Education

233) Word education is part of which constitutional list

a) State list since 1976

b) Concurrent list since 1947

c) Union list since 1936

d) Concurrent list since 1976

234) Algae blooms are ____ in oligotrophic lakes

a) More

b) Less

c) Very rare

d) Abundant

235) Identify the correct components of listening

a) Receive, understand, evaluate, isolate, respond

b) Receive, forward, evaluate, remember, respond

c) Receive, understand, evaluate, remember, respond

d) Receive, understand, evaluate, remember, repost

236) It is not a mass media effect theory

a) Positivism theory

b) Culturist theory

c) Class dominant theory

d) Limited effect theory

237) Complete the series

B, D, H, J, N, P, —

a) T

b) Y

c) W

d) Z

238) Proximal Development in Educational Communication was developed by

a) Akshapada gautama

b) Lev Vygotsky

c) Sigmund Freud

d) Philip Kotler

239) Complete the series 4,12,28,52, ___

a) 19

b) 67

c) 48

d) 84

e) 128

240) Latest update for B.Tech and B.E. Entrance Exam is ________

a) Entrance exam twice a year

b) No mandatory requirement of Maths and Physics in 12th

c) 1st year in B.Tech is study from home

d) Both B and C

241) With 5 books and 2 chapters in each book containing 528 aphoristic sutras. These are called

a) Kalpa sutra

b) Srauta sutra

c) Dharma sutra

d) Nyaya sutra

e) Grya sutra

f) Patanjali Sutra

242) Nyaya sutra was written by

a) Rishi Kannada

b) Rishi Vishwanath Prajapati

c) Rishi Patanjali

d) Rishi Akshapada Gautam

243) Match the following

LIST - 1 (Ind AS)	LIST - 2 (Titles)
A. Ind AS 102	1. Insurance contract
B. Ind AS 104	2. Share based payments
C. Ind AS 106	3. Operating segments
D. Ind AS 108	4. Exploration and evaluation of mineral resources.

1. A-1, B-2, C-3, D-4
2. A-2, B-1, C-4, D-3
3. A-4, B-1, C-3, D-2
4. A-2, B-1, C-4, D-3

244) Identify correct statements: -

a) According to Ind AS 101, first time adoption of Ind AS, has to be disclosed through income(P&L) statement.

b) Ind AS 103, business combination has to be recognized in financial statement jointly and separately for all the assets and liabilities of the combination.

c) Ind AS 105, non-current assets held for sale and discontinued from business have to be reported separately.

d) Ind AS 108, operating segments, for a group of companies have to be reported through segments of financial statements.

Choose the correct statements:

A) A, B, C

B) A, C, D

C) B, C, D

D) A, B, D

245) ABC Ltd. Has a PE ratio of 2.4 with MPS of Rs.87 and the firm has a DPR Ratio of 72%. Calculate dividend paid and EPS.

a) Rs.26.10, Rs.36.25.

b) Rs.76.10, Rs.36.25.

c) Rs.21.10, Rs.14.25.

d) Rs.34.10, Rs.28.67.

Explanation:

PE = MPS/EPS

2.4 = 87 / x -> X = 87 / 2.4 -> X = 36.25 (EPS)DPR =

DPS/EPS -> 0.72 = y/36.25 -> Y = 0.72 * 36.25 -> Y = 26.10 Rs.(DPS)

246) A Firm has Sales of Rs.15 Lac from total assets of Rs.9 Lac, with Equity issued for Rs.5 Lac. It has a ROE of 3.5. Calculate Net income and expenses.?

a) 12.76 Lac, 2.24 Lac

b) 12.51 Lac, 7.76 Lac

c) 11.67 Lac, 5.13 Lac

d) 9.45 Lac, 2.19 Lac.

Explanation:

ROE = [NI/Sales]*[Sales/TA]*[TA/Equity] -> 3.5 = [x/15]*[15/9]*[9/5]

3.5 = [x/15]*[1.67]*[1.8]

3.5 = [x/15]*[3.006]

[x/15] = 3.006/3.5 -> [x/15] = 0.8588 > X = 0.85 * 15 -> X = 12.76

Expenses = Sales - Net Income => 15 Lac - 12.76 Lac = 2.24 Lac.

247) ABC Ltd. Has total liability of Rs.10 Lac, with non-current assets of 4.60 Lac and current liability of 3.70 Lac. Calculate current ratio and quick ratio, given that the inventory in stock is of Rs.1.80 Lac.

(A) 1.45; 3.70

(B) 3.70; 0.97

(C) 1.45; 0.97

(D) 0.97; 1.45.

Explanation:

Total liabilities = Total Assets -> 10 Lac = 10 Lac

(Equity + Non-Current Liability + Current Liability) = (Non-Current Asset + Current Assets)

[(6.30 Lac)+3.70 Lac] = [4.60 Lac + 5.40 Lac]

CR = CA/CL = 5.40/3.70 =1.45

QR = [CA-I]/CL = [5.40-1.80]/3.70 = 0.97

248) ABC Ltd. Has a working capital turnover ratio 3.89, with working capital of Rs.689,500/-. Calculate Sales.

a) Rs.36,54,000/-

b) Rs.46,71000/-

c) Rs.31,25000/-

d) Rs.26,82,155/-

Explanation:

3.89 = x / [689500]

X = 689500 * 3.89= 26,82,155.

249) Which of the following statement(s) are correct:

STATEMENT I: According to Richard Cantillons' Economic Entrepreneurship Theory, an Entrepreneur plays the role of an economic destructor.

STATEMENT II: According to Richard Cantillon, an Entrepreneur plays the role of both of a producer and a exchanger.

STATEMENT III:- Max Weber has said a startup develops if an entrepreneur accepts the system of the society and establishes his business, along the taboos of the society.

STATEMENT IV: Max Weber in his theory of Sociological Entrepreneurship has said a startup develops if an entrepreneur wishes not to accept the system of the society and establishes his business as against the taboos of the society system.

a) I and III

b) II and III

c) I and IV

d) III and IV.

250) Which of the following statement(s) are incorrect:

STATEMENT I: A 'Second generation Entrepreneur' pass on their businesses to 'third generation entrepreneurs'.

STATEMENT II: The 'First generation Entrepreneurs' have handled or operated some other business.

STATEMENT III: A 'Second generation Entrepreneur' adopts business initiated by his previous generation.

STATEMENT IV: A hustler entrepreneur is the one who is successful in his business and has started through self-orientation and motivation.

a) I, II Only

b) III, IV Only.

c) I, IV Only.

d) II, III Only.

251) ANSWER WHETHER THE FOLLOWING STATEMENT(S) ARE CORRECT OR INCORRECT:

STATEMENT I: A 'First Generation Entrepreneur' is the one who when starts a business, it is transferred to his further generation(s) and this person has no business exposure before this venture.

STATEMENT II: 'Second Generation Entrepreneurs' are the ones who adopt the family lineage business which was usually started by their grandfather/forefathers.

a) Both STATEMENT I and STATEMENT II are correct.

b) Both STATEMENT I and STATEMENT II are incorrect.

c) STATEMENT I is correct and STATEMENT II is incorrect.

d) STATEMENT I is incorrect and STATEMENT II is correct.

252) Factors which increase the teaching capabilities

a) Using teaching aids

b) Using teaching methods and strategies

c) Working with college administration

d) Having wealthy husband or father

e) Putting your heart in developing learning curves

253) An organizational climate is based on

a) Best personalities of employees

b) Commitment to mission and vision by employees

c) Correct attitude and value system of employees towards company's stakeholders

d) Reduction in under table payments and insider trading

254) To become a successful teacher, you should focus on

a) Using best teaching aids

b) Doing MLT or ULT or RLT teaching as the case maybe

c) Focus on developing learning curves of the learners

d) Focus on Working with college administration

e) Engage in lecture method of teaching to offload maximum content to learners

255) Most important pollutant which should not be totally discontinued from earth is

a) Arsenic

b) Nitrogen dioxide

c) Solar energy

d) Carbon

e) Benzene

256) While writing a research proposal one thing can be skipped

a) Financial requirements

b) Research population and its relevance

c) Objective of research

d) Who will be benefitted from this research

e) None of the above

257) A teacher should focus on

a) Program outcomes

b) Teaching with HOTS-LOTS technique

c) Using teaching aids

d) All of the above

e) Behavioural changes in learners

258) Most important work for a researcher is

a) Drafting a ethical research proposal

b) Selection of samples from population without biases

c) Completing researches without any technical lapses

d) None of the above

e) All

259) The main objective of Higher Education Commission of India (HECI) super regulator is to

a) Remove UGC

b) Remove AICTE

c) Act as single body of governance for Education

d) Act as a single body of governance for Higher Education

260) Most important out of the following is

a) Benzene

b) Cadmium

c) Arsenic

d) Mercury

e) All of the above

f) None

261) While teaching in a classroom, a teacher must use teaching aids only to

a) Enhance visual effects of the content

b) To beautify the slides of the presentation

c) To develop and increase the learning outcomes of the session

d) To expand the knowledge horizon of learners

262) If a researcher plans to do scientific research, his primary requirements are

a) A research lab

b) A detailed assessment of research is to be carried on

c) A choice between which hypothesis test is better

d) A clear understanding of the population to send a research proposal

263) Inadequacy of working capital, poor and obsolete technology, non-availability of raw material, inadequate demand, erratic power supply, labour problems, poor management, inability to face competition. These are reasons of

a) Group conflict

b) Sickness in industry or organization

c) Government assistance

d) Industrial dispute

264) A tundra and taiga are regions known as

a) Ecosystem

b) Habitat

c) A biome

d) A lithosphere zone

265) How many steps of research are valid for a researcher out of the following

a) Hypothesis, Data collection tools, Sampling, Proposal, Data collection, Data analysis, MLA format

b) Hypothesis, Data collection tools, Sampling, doing bias, Data collection tools, Sampling, Data analysis, Report writing

c) Hypothesis, finding a financier, Sampling, Proposal, Data collection, Data analysis, Report writing

d) Hypothesis, Data collection tools, Sampling, Proposal, Data collection, Data analysis, Report writing

266) When doing a research, a researcher is careful about

a) Research design

b) Research analysis

c) Research question

d) Research hypothesis

e) All of the above

f) None

267) A teacher is most effective in teaching if he/she does not let ---- affect his/ her teaching

a) Students need for understanding the concept

b) Institution's Management

c) Use Various teaching aids and changes in them time to time as required

d) Less experience in subject domain of a learner

268) When a null hypothesis is rejected, the following is the criterion?

a) Because researcher wants to accept alternative hypothesis.

b) Because data fails to answer the null hypothesis significantly

c) Because null hypothesis is a quantitative set

d) Because null hypothesis if accepted is a type 2 error.

269) Researcher is keen to find out

a) Flaws in already done researches of self or others.

b) Explore hidden angles to assumptions

c) Analyse researches to review them for relevant literature

d) Understand angles to hypothetical situations

270) National Income Approach ignores which source of income

a) Organization revenue

b) Govt Direct Tax/Indirect Tax Revenue

c) Subsidy provided to organizations

d) Depreciation expense

e) None of the above

f) All

271) Teaching aptitude is seen in which of the following situations

a) A teacher does help learner in his / her homework.

b) A teacher is constantly improvising his learning skills through training

c) A teacher is constantly improvising his teaching skills through constant vigil of strategies

d) A teacher is keen to help pass the learners in their exams and keep giving them material/books

272) Most important in a researcher's career

a) Getting a JRF and being associated with a good organization.

b) To create readership through marketing strategies

c) To follow standardized procedures and code of ethics

d) To never as questions from respondents after taking their consent

273) Which of the following best describes fundamental research?

a) It adds to existing scientific knowledge

b) It can be done easily

c) It does not require variable manipulation

d) It is field work-based research

274) Income approach does not include

a) Wages, Salary, Rent, Tax Revenue, Depreciation

b) Wages, Fixed Deposits made, Rent, Profits, Tax Revenue, Depreciation

c) Wages, Rent, Company Profits, Tax Revenue, Depreciation

d) Salary, Rent, Company Profits, Tax Revenue, Depreciation

275) According to Rudi Dornbusch in 1976, the foreign exchange rates react to changes in _____, to compensate for any types of sticky price based good within the economy.

a) Fiscal Policy

b) Economic Policy

c) Monetary Policy

d) All of the above.

276) Which of the following statement(s) are correct:

a. A successor activity with 0 free float starts 14th minute, if predecessor activity with total float is of 13 minutes.

b. The early start of a successor activity is the early finish of predecessor activity + free float.

c. The latest finish time of an activity is inclusive of its latest start time and total time taken to complete the activity.

A, B.

B, C.

A, C.

All of the above.

277) Which of the following statement(s) are incorrect:

a) A multivariate function depends on multiple input variables to produce an output.

b) A multivariate function is static at a given point.

c) Multivariate function deals with functions of several variables, leading to a single observation.

d) Multivariate function has its input made up of multiple numbers.

a) A Only.

b) B and C Only.

c) A and D Only.

d) B Only.

278) 6 % Expenditure of National Income is

a) National Policy, 1986

b) Kothari Commission, 1976

c) National Policy, 2020

d) National Policy, 1968

e) None of the above

279) EBIT- 15,34,600, EBT-7,12,400, Debt - ? FL -?

a) 8,12,640,2.34

b) 8,23,200,1.15

c) 8,22,200, 2.15

d) None of the above.

280) BIOS is

a) Basic Inverted output software

b) Boolean Input Output System

c) Basic Input Output System

d) Bas in ——

281) Job analysis is most important

a) Activity before making job evaluation/recruitment

b) Activity before making job description

c) Activity before making job analysis

d) Activity before job recruitment.

282) Researchers are

a) Studious

b) Keep an eye for detail

c) Fond of books

d) All of the above

283) Most non-innovative is

a) Manager

b) Leader

c) Fabian/Drone

284) The Great Indian Bustard is found in

a) Kaizaranga National Park

b) Thar Desert, Rajasthan

c) Gir Forests

d) Nonsense

285) If T is a proposition, its contradictory is

a) Undetermined

b) True

c) False

d) Nonsense

286) Ecology is of

a) 3 types

b) Study of land

c) Study of animals

d) Study of flowers

287) Identify the factors that affect teaching

a) Teaching methods chosen

b) Use of blackboard only

c) Strategies to teach

d) Economic environment of the country

e) Example based teaching

SOLUTION:

a) a,b,c

b) b,c,e

c) a,c,e

d) All of the above

288) Classroom effectiveness requires which of the following

a) Use of Teaching Aids

b) Use of ICT

c) Group communication

d) Teaching skills

e) Setting more and more homework

1. A, B, C

2. B, D, E

3. A, C, E

4. A, B, C, D

289) For fund flow statements, which of the following statement is incorrect?

a) Records 2 types of transactions: Sources and application of funds?

b) Issues of debentures - sources of funds

c) Land brought- application of funds

d) Salaries paid – Application of funds

e) All of the above

f) None of the above

290) Which of the following is true for National Education Polic for India?

a) 1968- Distance Education System

b) 2020- Name of MHRD changed to Ministry of Education

c) 1986- National Income Expenditure allowed on Education

d) All of the above

e) None

291) Banks while giving loans should take care of which of the following:

a) Promoters should have invested there at least some capital in the company F

b) There should be some minimal fixed/current assets with the company. True

292) GHG is a part of which 2 countries agreement

a) Montreal + Kyoto

b) Kyoto + Paris

c) Montreal+ Ramsar

d) SDG+ MDG

293) Increase/Decrease of flow of FDI in/out of country will result in

a) Inc/Dec of current account

b) Inc/Dec of FDI account

c) Inc/Dec of financial Account

d) Inc/Dec of Balance of Payments account

294) INDC are submitted by member countries every 5 years under

a) Montreal protocol

b) Convention on biodiversity

c) Paris accord

d) International Solar Alliance

295) OTM call option will have a strike price that is higher than the market price of the underlying asset.

a) Correct

b) Incorrect

296) A research company collects data through some college students. This method of collection is called

a) Primary data

b) Secondary data

c) Primary source data collection

d) Secondary source data collection

297) Cash flow of issued common stock of Rs 10 L

a) Inflow (+), Investing activity

b) Outflow (-), Financing activity

c) Outflow (-), Investing activity

d) Inflow (+), Financing activity

298) SWAYAM is portal for

a) Promoting high quality education

b) Improving access to high quality education

c) Telecasting high quality educational content free of charge

d) Both b and c

299) What is the difference between interval/ratio and ordinal variables?

a) The distance between categories is equal to across the range of interval/ ratio data.

b) Ordinal data can be rank ordered but interval/ratio data cannot

c) Interval / ratio variables contain only 2 categories

d) Ordinal variables have a fixed zero point where as interval/ratio variables do not

300) Identify Paanch Mahaviraas

a) Vikramshila, Nalanda, Somapura, Odantapura, Jagaddala

b) Vikramshila, Nalanda, Somapura, Takshila, Jagaddala

c) Vajrayana, Takshila, Somapura, Odantapuri, Jagaddala

d) Vikramshila, Nalanda, Somapura, Vajrayana, Jagaddala

Answer Key Mock Test - 3

201) a) Market Linked Focus Product Scheme
202) e) Both A, C
203) d) AOA
204 d) Research Process
205 g) Unnat Bharat Vaccine
206 a) Aspirant-> Performer-> Front Runner-> Achiever
207 d) Kerela and Chandigarh
208 2) B and C
209 b) Angadwadi
210 b) Academic Council
211 b) Regulations+ Education + Research+ Grants+ Accreditation
212 c) Regulations
213 c) Ashtadhyayi
214 b) Miranda House> Lady Shri Ram College > Loyola College
215 d) Dr. B.R. Ambedkar Univesity, 1982
216 a) MM's approach to dividend
217 d) Research Epistemology
218 d) Retained Earnings + Promoters Capital+ Deferred expenses
219 d) Getting good and dedicated staff
220 d) Residential area + Nuclear plant
221 d) While highlighting key points
222 c) A-III, B-II C-I
223 b) A-II, B-III, C-I
224 d) Carbon Sink
225 d) 33-35 % of GDP
226 c) Biodiversity
227 c) Snowball sampling
228 d) Lokayata and Kapalika
229 b) 2 only
230 a) Inductive argument
231 c) Some apricots are real
232 d) CABE
233 d) Concurrent list since 1976
234 c) Very rare
235 c) Receive, understand, evaluate, remember, respond
236 a) Positivism theory
237 a) True
238 b) Lev Vygotsky
239 d) 84
240 b) No mandatory requirement of Maths and Physics in 12th
241 d) Nyaya sutra
242 d) Rishi Akshapada Gautam
243 A-2, B-1, C-4, D-3
244 B, C, D
245 a. Rs.26.10, Rs.36.25.
246 a. 12.76 Lac, 2.24 Lac
247 c) 1.45; 0.97
248 a. Rs.26,82,155/-
249 b) II and III
250 a) I and II Only.
251 c) STATEMENT I is correct and STATEMENT II is incorrect.
252 e) Putting your heart in developing learning curves
253 c) Correct attitude and value system of employees.
254 c) Focus on developing learning curves of the learners
255 d) Carbon
256 e) None of the above
257 e) Behavioural changes in learners
258 e) All
259 d) Act as a single body of governance for Higher Education
260 f) None
261 c) To develop and increase the learning outcomes of the session
262 b) A detailed assessment of research is to be carried on
263 b) Sickness in industry or organization
264 c) a biome
265 d) Hypothesis, Data collection tools, Sampling, Proposal, Data collection, Data analysis, Report writing
266 e) All of the above
267 d) Less experience in subject domain of a learner
268 b) Because data fails to answer the null hypothesis significantly
269 c) analyse researches to review them for relevant literature

270 c) Subsidy provided to organizations
271 c) A teacher is constantly improvising his teaching skills through constant vigil of strategies
272 c) To follow standardized procedures and code of ethics
273 d) It is field work-based research
274 b) Wages, Fixed Deposits made, Rent, Profits, Tax Revenue, Depreciation
275 C
276 B
277 D
278 d) National Policy, 1968
279 c) 8,22,200, 2.15
280 c) Basic Input Output System
281 b) Activity before making job description
282 d) All of the above
283 c) Fabian/Drone
284 b) Thar Desert, Rajasthan
285 c) False
286 a) 3 types (autecology, synecology, and ecosystem ecology)
287 C) a,c,e
288 A, B, C, D
289 f) None of the above
290 b) 2020- Name of MHRD changed to Ministry of Education
291 False, True
292 b) Kyoto + Paris
293 c) Inc/Dec of financial Account
294 c) Paris accord
295 a) Correct
296 c) Primary source data collection
297 d) Inflow (+), Financing activity
298 d) Both b and c
299 a) The distance between categories is equal to across the range of interval/ratio data.
300 a) Vikramshila, Nalanda, Somapura, Odantapura, Jagaddala

Practice Mock Test - 4

301) How might quantitative research help qualitative research?

a) By identifying specific groups of people to be interviewed

b) By utilizing a rigorous positivist framework

c) By combining laboratory experiments with structured participant observation

d) By showing the occurrence of different responses to a survey

302) In an experimental design, the dependent variable is

a) The one that is not manipulated and in which any changes are observed

b) The one that is manipulated in order to observe any effects on the other.

c) A measure of the extent to which personal values affect research

d) An ambiguous concept whose meaning depends on how it is defined.

303) The standard error is a statistical measure of

a) Normal distribution of scores around the mean sample

b) Extent to which a sample is likely to differ from the population mean

c) Clustering of scores at each end of a survey scale

d) Degree to which a sample has been accurately stratified

304) ----- on capital is called Cost of Capital

a) Lower expected return

b) Normally expected return

c) Higher expected return

d) None of the above

305) Consider a graph with standard deviation on the horizontal axis and expected return on the vertical axis. The line that connects the risk-free rate and the optimal risky portfolio is called

a) The security market line

b) The capital market line

c) The indifference curve

d) The characteristic line

306) Which cost is not considered during the calculations of cost sheet ?

a) Factory cost

b) Goodwill written off

c) Labour cost

d) Selling cost

307) Find out the leverage ratio if the capital structure has Rs 4,00,000 equity and Rs 1,60,000 debt

a) 29%

b) 28.57%

c) 24%

d) 67%

308) The traditional approach towards the valuation of a company assumes that ------

a) The cost of capital is independent of the capital structure of the firm

b) Management can increase the total value of the firm through judicious use of financial leverage

c) The firm maintains constant risk regardless of the type of financing employed.

d) There exists no optimal structure

309) One assumption underlying the use of the cost of capital to analyze capital projects is that

a) Current costs will remain the same

b) Capital structure will vary with the type of financing

c) Different risks projects are required to diversify the firm

d) The analysed projects are of comparable risk to existing projects

310) In calculating the costs of the individual components of a firm's financing, the corporate tax rate is important to which of the following component cost formulas?

a) Equity stock

b) Debentures

c) Preferred equity stock

d) Company deposits

311) Which of the following is an example of deception in business research?

a) Obtaining of company material without permission

b) Researcher wearing a disguise during an observation

c) Researcher representing their research as being about a different topic

d) Researcher failing to ask permission to interview someone.

312) The scale applied in statistics which imparts a difference of magnitude and proportions is considered as

a) Exponential scale

b) Ratio Scale

c) Goodness scale

d) Satisfactory scale

313) The variables whose calculation is done according to the weight, height and length and weight are known as

a) Flowchart variables

b) Discrete variables

c) Continuous variables

d) Measuring variables

314) A numerical value used as a summary measure for a sample such as ample mean is known as

a) Population parameter

b) Sample parameter

c) Sample statistic

d) Population mean

315) Amit bought 5 kg rice for Rs 1420 and sold 2 kg rice for Rs 460.Find out profit or loss

a) Loss Rs 74

b) Profit Rs 230

c) Loss Rs 54

d) Profit Rs 284

316) A general rule for managers to follow is to set the firms capital structure such that

a) Firm's value is minimized

b) Firms value is maximized

c) Firms' bondholders are made well off

d) Firm's suppliers of raw materials are satisfied

e) Firm's dividend payout is maximized

317) The proposition that the cost of equity isa positive linear function of capital structure is called

a) The capital asset pricing model

b) MM proposition I

c) MM proposition II

d) The efficient markets hypothesis

318) A firm or an individual or a Hindu Undivided Family (HUF) whose books of account are required to be audited under section 44 B shall furnish the return of income electronically under digital signature.

a) True

b) False

319) Arrange the following parties in sequence in the event dissolution of a firm

1) Secured creditors

2) Unsecured creditors

3) Partners who have granted loans

4) Partners who contributed over and above pro-sharing ratio

a) 2,1,3,4

b) 1,2,3,4

c) 1,2,4,3

d) 2,1,4,3

320) Which of the following is not ensured to the consumer in case of globalization?

a) A and B

b) A and C

c) B and C

d) C and D

321) Emotional intelligence of learners

322) Standard quantity 40 kg, Standard Rate Rs 2/kg, Actual Cost Rs 90 and actual rate Rs 3/kg. Calculate Material Cost Variance and Material Usage Variance

a) 10(A), 20(F)

b) 10(F), 20(F)

c) 10(F), 20(A)

d) 15(A), 28(F)

323) The Indian banking system consists of ___ public sector banks, ___ private sector banks, ____ foreign banks, ____ regional rural banks, ____ rural cooperative banks + cooperative credit institutions.

a) 20,22,44,44,1542,94000

b) 20,22,44,44,1542,94384

c) 20,22,44,44,15000, 94384

d) 20,000, 22,24, 44000,1542,94384

324) A single overall cost of capital is often used to evaluate projects because

a) It avoids the problem of computing the rate of return for each investment proposal.

b) It is the only way to measure a firm's required return.

c) It acknowledges that most new investment projects have about the same degree of risk.

325) Effectiveness of teaching?

a) Marks obtained by students in overall subjects.

b) Level of realization of instructional objectives

c) Time taken by the students to learn

d) Resources used by the teacher in teaching

a) (a), (A), (b) and (C)

b) (b), (A), (B) and (D)

c) (c), (B), (C) AND (D)

326) A company's bank account has a credit from Reliance Ltd, for its preference equity held. Suggest its entry in A company financial statement- cash flow and flow statements.

a) Investing activity, application of fund

b) Investing activity, sources of fund

c) Financing activity, sources of fund

d) Financing activity, application of fund

327) Which one of the following would be considered a protective strategy ?

a) Buy a put on a stock you own

b) Sell a call against a stock you sold short

c) Sell a put on a stock you own

d) Buy a call on a stock you own

e) Sell a naked put.

328) The difference between the value of a call option and aput option with the same exercise price is primarily due to

a) Volatility of the price of the underlying

b) The greater liquidity of call options

c) Use of continuous as opposed to discrete discounting.

d) Effect of dividends on the two securities

e) The differential between the current stock price and the exercise price in present value terms.

329) How might qualitative research assist with the analysis of quantitative data?

a) By providing statistical data

b) By identifying a sample of respondents for triangulation

c) By making the research more value-laden and subjective

d) By assisting the explanation of the relationship between 2 variables

330) How might quantitative research support qualitative research?

a) By identifying specific groups of people to be interviewed

b) By utilizing a rigorous positivist framework

c) By combining laboratory experiments with structured participant obersvation

331) What is one of the main ethical problems associated with conducting a secondary analysis of qualitative data?

a) The participants may not have given informed consent to the res use of their data.

b) It involves deceiving respondents about the nature of the research.

c) The secondary analyst must adopt a covert role and is at risk of going native.

d) Respondents are likely to experience physical harm as a result of the process.

332) Why should you stat coding your data as soon as possible?

a) To sharpen your focus and help with theoretical sampling

b) Because researchers always run out of time at the end of a project

c) Because it is the easiest thing to do

d) To make sure that your initial theoretical ideas are imposed on the data

333) The standard error is a statistical measure of:

a) The normal distribution around the sample mean
b) The extent to which a sample mean is likely to differ from the population mean
c) The clustering of scores at each end of a survey score
d) The degree to which a sample has been acutely stratified

334) A simple random sample is one in which

a) From a random starting point, every nth unit from the sampling frame is selected.
b) A non-probability strategy is used making the results difficult to generalize
c) The researcher has a certain quota of respondents to fill for various social groups
d) Every unit of the population has an equal chance of being selected.

335) Complete the following series

(A) 2,5,11,23,47, 95?
(B) 5,16, 65?
(C) 5,4,7,20, 79?
(a) 191,346,396
(b) 191,326,394
(c) Mera....

336) Which of the following are sampling considerations?

a) Who do you want to study in order to investigate your research questions?
b) How easily can you gain access to a sampling frame?
c) What kind of sampling strategy will you employee?
d) All the above

337) What practical steps can you take before you actually start your research?

a) Find out exactly whatever your institutions requirements are?
b) Make sure you are familiar with the hardware and software that you want to use?
c) Apply for clearance of your project through a clearance committee
d) All the above

338) A measure of internal consistency – how closely related as a set of items ae as a group. It is considered to be a measure of scale reliability.

a) Jensen Alpha
b) Cronbach Alpha
c) Both a and B

339) When research subjects are given slightly different questions or measures of the same concept to help increase the reliability of the research results, this is referred to as

a) Intra-observer reliability
b) Interitem reliability
c) Intercoder reliability
d) Alternate forms reliability

340) A goal of some researcher's is to be able to generalize their findings to the larger population. This is referred to as

a) Internal validity
b) External validity
c) Operationalization
d) Cronbach Alpha

341) If 2 researchers study the same subject yet record (enter into the data analysis software) 2 different responses, this is referred to as

a) Intra observer reliability

b) Interitem reliability

c) Intercoder reliability

d) Alternate forms reliability

342) The research term indicating that unknown variables maybe influencing the relationship between the independent and dependent variable is known as

a) Exogenous variables

b) Outlier variables

c) Predictor variables

d) None of the above

343) What is meant when the term co-vary is used in research methods?

a) As one variable changes so does the other variable

b) Result research depends on the varying qualities of the researcher skills

c) If 2 researchers achieve the same research results, they are said to co-vary

d) None of the above

344) Which of the following should be included in a research proposal?

a) Your academic status and experience

b) The difficulties that you encountered with our previous reading on the topic

c) Your choice of research methods and reasons for choosing them

d) All of the above

345) Ram travels with a speed of 40 km/hr. If he has to travel a distance of 740 km, how much time will he take

a) 19 min

b) 18.5 hours

c) 19 hours

d) 25 min

346) Current market price share is Rs 150. Dividend is Rs 25. Cost of equity capital is 10%. Find the new MPS

a) 158

b) 148

c) 140

d) 210

347) Average Salary of Amit and Sumit is 15,860. Salary of Sumit is 21,000. Find out the salary of Amit?

a) 15000

b) 10,720

c) 21,550

d) 15,485

348) Which of the following requirements for a dissertation may depend on your institution?

a) Whether an abstract should be included?

b) The format for referencing

c) Size of the study

d) All of the above

349) Consumer can obtain information from any of several sources like information from handling, examining or using product then consumer would have obtained the information by usin

a) Personal source

b) Commercial source

c) Informative source

d) Experiential source

350) Survey research is cross-sectional and as a result it is

a) Low in internal validity but high in replicability

b) High in internal validity but low in reliability

c) None of the above

d) High in ecological validity but low in external validity

351) Section that gives various items on which tax is to be collected at source is

a) 201

b) 203 A

c) 203AA

d) 206C

352) To say that the forward market lacks equidity means that

a) Forward contracts usually result in losses

b) Forward contracts cannot be turned into cash

c) It may be difficult to make the transaction

d) None of the above

353) Which of the following should you think about when preparing your research?

a) Your sample frame and sampling strategy

b) The ethical issues that might arise

c) Negotiating access to the setting

d) All the above

354) By selling short a futures contract of Rs. 1,00,000 at a price of 115 you are agreeing to deliver

a) Rs 1,00,000 face value securities for Rs 1,15,000

b) Rs 1,15,000 face value securities for Rs 1,10,000

c) Rs 1,00,000 face value securities for Rs 1,00,000

d) Rs 1,15,000 face value securities for Rs 1,15,000

355) A long contract requires that the investor

a) Sells securities in the future

b) Buy the security in the future

c) Hedge in the future

d) Close out his position in the future

356) The term 'external' validity is concerned with

a) Whether results of a study can be generalized beyond specific research context

b) By whether the research question is judge to be a good research question by those outside the study

c) Whether social scientific findings are applicable to people's every day, natural social settings.

d) An ambiguous concept whose meaning depends on how it is defined

357) Which of the following is not a feature of ethics in research?

a) A researcher collects data for institute without approval of research proposal.

b) A researcher asks personal questions from respondents

c) A researcher prepares a research design before data collection

d) A researcher draws samples put of population to conduct this research.

e) All of the above

f) None

358) Why is it more important to have well formulated research questions?

a) Gives greater clarity to the research process and what you wish to research

b) It leads to more focussed research

c) It provides more structure to my work

d) All of the above

359) What is research design?

a) A way of conducting research that is not grounded in theory.

b) The choice between using qualitative and quantitative methods

c) The style in which you present your research findings eg. A graph

d) A framework for every stage of the collection and analysis of data.

360) A statement whose validity is tested on the basis of a sample is called

a) Null hypothesis

b) Statistical hypothesis

c) Simple hypothesis

d) Composite hypothesis

361) Communication with oneself is called

a) Organizational

b) Grapevine

c) Interpersonal

d) Intrapersonal

362) The point where the null hypothesis gets rejected is called

a) Significant value

b) Rejection value

c) Acceptance value

d) Critical value

363) By which of the following proposition, the proposition, some men are not honest is contradicted.

a) All men are honest

b) Some men are honest

c) No men are honest

d) All of the above

364) Internal validity refers to

a) Whether or not there is a casual relationship between 2 variables

b) Whether or not the findings are relevant to researcher's everyday lives.

c) The extent to which the researcher believes that this was a worthwhile project

d) How accurately the measurements represent underlying concepts

365) The primary duty of the teacher is to

a) Raise the intellectual standard of the students

b) Improve the physical standard of the students

c) Help all round development of the students

d) Imbibe value system in the students

366) When subject and predicate of both the premises are same but they differ in quality only, it is known as

a) Contradictories

b) Contraries

c) Subaltern

d) Superaltern

367) Budgeted overheads- Rs 2,55,000. Overhead rate was pre-decided at Rs 5.1per labour hours, actual 52,000 instead of 51,000 hours. Actual overheads resulted in a rate of Rs 4.9 labour hours. Volume variance is

a) Rs 5100 favourable

b) Rs 5200 favourable

c) Rs 5100 unfavourable

d) Rs 5200 unfavourable

368) A deductive argument is invalid if

a) It's premises and conclusion are all false

b) It's premises are all false but conclusion is true

c) It's premises are all true but conclusion is false

d) It's premises and conclusion are all true

369) Name the scheme which facilitates academic and research collaboration between Indian institution and best institution in the world

a) ICSSR-IMPRESS

b) Sta Development Scheme

c) Institutional Development Scheme

d) SPARC

370) Assertion: There are more laws on the books today than ever before and more crimes being committed than ever before.

Reason: Because to reduce crime we must eliminate the laws.

a) A is true, R is doubtful and R is not the correct explanation of A

b) A is false R is true and R is the correct explanation of A

c) A is doubtful, R is doubtful and R is not the correct explanation of A

d) A is doubtful, R is true and R is not the correct explanation of A

371) Introducing Rakesh to her husband a woman said, "His brother's father is the only son of my grandfather. The woman is related to Rakesh as:

a) Aunt

b) Mother

c) Sister

d) Daughter

372) Montreal protocol aims at

a) Reduction in emission of green-house gases

b) Phasing out ozone depleting substances

c) Prohibiting transboundary movement of hazardous waste

d) Enhancing cooperation among UN member states for peaceful uses of nuclear energy

373) According to the analysis of the British economist John Mayard Keynes

a) Markets coordinate supply and demand so that a policy of laissez-faire would prevent recessions

b) Economic fluctuations - cumulative result of mistakes made by business, households in uncertainty.

c) Government demand could be used to smooth fluctuations in aggregate output and income

d) Supply creates its own demand through the circular flow of economic activity

374) The set of computer programs that manage the hardware/software of a computer is called

a) Compiler system

b) Operation system

c) Operating system

d) None of these

375) The long run average cost scale

a) Is constructed using short run marginal cost curves

b) Is an upside-down U Shaped

c) Slows economies and diseconomies of scale

d) Both A and B

e) Both A and C

376) Mass media do not have pre - determined functions for everyone and people use them the way they like. This is suggestive of the fact that

a) Audiences are active

b) Content is of little significance

c) Content lacks plurality

d) Audiences are homogenous

377) The value of money supports the comparison of cash flows recorded at different time period by

a) Discounting all cash flows to a common point of time

b) Compounding all cash flows to a common point of time

c) Either a or b

d) None of the above

378) gif, jpg, bmp, png are used as extensions for files which store

a) Image data

b) Audio Data

c) Video Data

d) Text Data

379) A current asset that can be transferred into cash within 3 months is known as

a) Cash equivalent

b) Intangible asset

c) Operating asset

d) Cash Asset

380) Which of the following is an example of a circular agreement?

a) God created man in his image and man created God in his own image

b) God is the source of a scripture and the scripture is the source of our knowledge of God

c) Some of The Indians are great because India is great

d) Rama is great because he is Rama

381) Which of the following would be consistent with an aggressive approach to financing working capital?

a) Financing short terms needs with short term funds

b) Financing permanent inventory build-up with long term debt

c) Financing seasonal needs with short term funds

d) Financing some long-term needs with short term funds

382) Main functions of UGC:

1) Recognition of institutions

2) Maintenance of quality and standards

3) Appointment of Vice Chancellor

4) Giving grants to institutions

5) Making state governments responsible for educational development

A. 1, 2, 3.

B. 1, 4, 5

C. 1, 2, 4

D. 2, 3, 5

383) 2 statements are related in such a way that one becomes undetermined, other will also be undetermined

a) Every fruit is nutritious

b) Fruits are hardly nutritious

c) Fruits are mostly nutritious

d) Some food items are nutritious

1. A and B Only

2. B and C Only

3. C and D Only

4. A and D Only

384) A deductive argument cannot be valid:

a) If its premise/premises is / are true and its conclusion is true

b) If its premise/premises is / are true and its conclusion is false

c) If its premise/premises is / are false and its conclusion is false

d) If its premise/premises is / are true and its conclusion is true

385) Jennifer's father-in-law is my brother. Helen is grand-daughter of my mother. How is Helen related to Jennifer?

a) Daughter in Law

b) Sister

c) Sister-in-Law

d) Mother

386) If the demand curve for a firms output is perfectly elastic , then the firm is

a) A monopolist

b) Perfectly competitive

c) An oligopolistic

d) A monopolistically competitive

387) Find analogy: 7:13: 9?

a) 8

b) 9

c) 7

d) 6

388) Find analogy:

a) 36

b) 100

c) 121

d) 144

389) Which of the following is not a matter of global concern in the removal of tropical forests?

a) Their ability to absorb the chemicals that could contribute to depletion of ozone layer

b) Their role in maintaining the oxygen and carbon balance of the earth

c) The ability to regulate surface and air temperatures, moisture content and reflectivity

d) Their contribution to the biological diversity of the planet

390) a) All poets are philosophers

b) Some poets are philosophers

c) Some poets are not philosophers

d) No philosopher is a poet

a) b & c

b) a & b

c) a & d

d) a & c

391) If a good is normal then a decrease in price will cause a substitution effect that is

a) Positive and an income effect that is positive

b) Positive and an income effect that is negative

c) Negative and an income effect that is positive

d) Negative and an income effect that is negative

392) Picture on direction sense test

a) Facing south west

b) Facing east

c) Facing west

d) Facing south

e) Facing north west

393) An individual stork required return is equal to risk free rate plus bearing risk premium is an explanation of

a) Security market line'

b) Capital market line'

c) Aggregate market line

d) Beta market line

394) It production started in 1965, today the world's government wants to get rid of it. This act of elimination is celebrated as

a) International Teacher's Day

b) Teachers Day. 5th Sept

c) World Environment Day, 2022

d) International Plastic Bag Free Day, 3rd July

395) Which of the following statements about classical economists in the 19th century is false?

a) They used the term trade cycles, not business cycles

b) They knew cycles existed because of fluctuations in measured real GDP

c) They believed that the typical cycle lasted between seven and eleven years

d) They suggested that one cause of cycles was the activity of sunspots on the sun.

396) The betas that tend to move towards 1.0 with the passage of time are classified as

a) Standard betas

b) Varied betas

c) Historical betas

d) Adjusted betas

397) The negative minimum risk portfolio of any security shows that market security sold is

a) Less than original price

b) Greater than original price

c) Equal to original price

d) Equal to sum of stocks

398) Which of these is not an effective commandant of effective communication?

a) Clarity in language

b) Poor listening

c) Home communication

d) Adequate medium

399) A reasoning where we start with certain particular statements and conclude with a universal statement is called

a) Deductive reasoning

b) Inductive reasoning

c) Abnormal reasoning

d) Transcendental reasoning

400) If a large diamond is cut into little bits it will lose its value just as an army us divided into small units of soldiers, It loses its strengths. The argument put above maybe called as

a) Analogical

b) Deductive

c) Statistical

d) Casual

Answer Key Mock Test - 4

301 a) By identifying specific groups of people to be interviewed
302 a) The one that is not manipulated and in which any changes are observed
303 b) Extent to which a sample is likely to differ from the population mean
304 b) Normally expected return
305 b) The capital market line
306 b) Goodwill written off
307 b) 28.57 %
308 b) Management can increase the total value of the firm
309 c) Different risks projects are required to diversify the firm
310 b) Debentures
311 c) Researcher representing their research about different topic
312 b) Ratio Scale
313 c) Continuous variables
314 c) Sample statistic
315 c) Loss Rs 54
316 b) Firms value is maximized
317 c) MM proposition II
318 a) True
319 c) 1,2,4,3
320 c) B and C
321 Emotional intelligence of learners
322 a) 10(A), 20(F)
323 b) 20,22,44,44,1542,94384
324 a) It avoids computing the ROR for each investment proposal.
325 a) (a), (A), (b) and (C)
326 b) Investing activity, sources of fund
327 a) Buy a put on a stock you own
328 e) Differential -current stock price & exercise price in present value
329 d) By assisting explanation of relationship between two variables.
330 a) By identifying specific groups of people to be interviewed
331 a) Participants have not given informed consent.
332 d) To make sure that initial theoretical ideas are imposed on data
333 b) Extent to which a sample mean differs from population mean
334 d) Every unit of population has an equal chance of being selected.
335 (b) 191,326,394
336 d) All the above
337 d) All the above
338 b) Cronbach Alpha
339 d) Alternate form's reliability
340 b) External validity
341 c) Intercoder reliability
342 a) Exogenous variables
343 a) As one variable change so does the other variable
344 c) Your choice of research methods and reasons for choosing them
345 b) 18.5 hours
346 c) 140
347 b) 10,720
348 d) All of the above
349 d) Experiential source
350 a) Low in internal validity but high in replicability
351 d) 206C
352 c) It may be difficult to make the transaction
353 d) All the above
354 a) Rs 1,00,000 face value securities for Rs 1,15,000
355 b) Buy the security in the future
356 a) Whether results of study are generalized beyond specific context
357 e) All of the above
358 d) All of the above
359 d) A framework for every stage of collection and analysis of data.
360 b) Statistical hypothesis
361 d) Intrapersonal
362 d) Critical value
363 a) All men are honest
364 a) Whether or not there is a casual relationship between 2 variables

365 c) Help all round development of the students
366 b) Contraries
367 a) Rs 5100 favourable
368 c) Its premises are all true but conclusion is false
369 d) SPARC
370 a) A is true, R is doubtful and R is not the correct explanation of A
371 c) Sister
372 b) Phasing out ozone depleting substances
373 c) Government demand used to smooth fluctuations in aggregate output & income
374 c) Operating system
375 c) Slows economies and diseconomies of scale
376 a) Audiences are active
377 c) Either a or b
378 a) Image data
379 a) Cash equivalent
380 b) God is source of scripture which is source of knowledge of God
381 d) Financing some long-term needs with short term funds
382 C. 1, 2, 4
383 1. A and B Only
384 b) If its premise/premises is / are true and its conclusion is false
385 c) Sister-in-Law
386 b) Perfectly competitive
387 b) 9
388 b) 100
389 a) Ability to absorb chemicals contributing to depletion of ozone layer
390 d) a and c
391 a) Positive and an income effect that is positive
392 d) Facing south
393 a) Security market line'
394 d) International Plastic Bag Free Day, 3rd July
395 b) Cycles existed because of fluctuations in measured real GDP
396 d) Adjusted betas
397 a) Less than original price
398 b) Poor listening
399 b) Inductive reasoning
400 a) Analogical

Practice Mock Test - 5

401) General reserves opening and closing balance Rs 10,000 and Rs 9000. Additional information- loss of Rs 1000 has been written off in general reserves. Decline in reserve and loss on investment adjusted in P&L account

a) True

b) False

402) Which is the statements is logically valid?

a) Most teachers are hardworking

Conclusions: 1) Some teachers are hardworking 2) Some teachers are not hard working.

a) Only I is implied

b) Only II is implied

c) Both I and II are implied

d) Neither I and II are implied

403) Research ethics has a direct connection more often with which stage of research

a) Defining and delimiting the scope of research

b) Problem formulation and reporting of research findings

c) Defining the population and deciding the sampling technique for research

d) Deciding the statistical techniques and data analysis

404) IF A is coded as C, M as I, N as P, S as 0, I as A, P as N, E as M, 0 as E and C as S then the code of COMPANIES will be

a) SPEINMOAC

b) NCPSEIOMA

c) SMOPIEACN

d) SEIN CPAMO

405) Liquid assets are determined by

a) Current assets-stock-Prepaid expenses

b) Current assets + stock + Prepaid expenses

c) Current assets + Prepaid expenses

d) None of the above

406) While calculating cash flow from operating activities which of the following will be deducted

a) Decrease in prepaid expenses

b) Increase in trade payables

c) Increase in trade receivables

d) Decrease in trade receivables

407) ASSERTION: Classroom communication has a cultural dimension.

REASON: Beliefs, habits, customs and languages are the cultural characteristics of communication

a) Both (A) & (R) are true and (R) is the correct explanation of A

b) Both (A) & (R) are true but (R) is not the correct explanation of A

(c) (A) is true but (R) is false

(d) (A) is false but (R) is true

408) The proposition that the value of a levered firm is equal to the value of an unlevered firm is known as

a) MM proposition I with no tax

b) MM proposition II with no tax

c) MM proposition I with tax

d) MM proposition II with tax

e) State theory proposition

409) THE UGC-MANDATE 2020 Scheme for trans - disciplinary research grants is

a) SATAT

b) STRIDE

c) SOCIAL AND INDUSTRY CONNECT

d) Consortium for Academic and Research Ethics (CARE)

410) The change in firm value in the presence of corporate taxes only is

a) Positive as equity holders face a lower effective tax rate

b) Positive as equity holders gain the tax shield on the debt interest

c) Negative because of the increased risk of default and fewer shares outstanding

d) Negative because of the reduction in equity outstanding

411) Price earnings Ratio

a) Market Price per share /Earnings per share

b) Earnings per share / Market Price per share

c) (Market Price per share X no of shares) / Earnings per share

d) Market Price per share/ (Earnings per share X no of shares)

412) Four major operations in scientific research are

a) Demonstration of co-variance

b) Elimination of spurious relations

c) Sequencing in terms of time order

d) Self-education

e) Operationalization of personal choice

f) Theorization

1) a, b, c, d

2) c, d, e, f

3) a, b, c, f

4) b, c, d, e

413) A firm should select the capital structure which

a) Produces the highest cost of capital

b) Maximises the value of the firm

c) Minimizes taxes

d) Is fully unlevered

e) Has no debt

414) Physical geography studies the results of the interaction between man and nature in order to

a) Understand global climate change

b) Study the impact of man's activities on nature

c) Address the issue of global climate change

d) Reduce man animal conflict

415) House tax savings of the firm derived from the deductibility of interest expenses is called the

a) Interest tax shield

b) Depreciable shield

c) Financing umbrella

d) Current yield

e) Tax-loss carry forward savings

416) The initial efforts for internet-based communication were for

a) Commercial communication

b) Military purposes

c) Personal interaction

d) Political campaigns

417) Financial leverage amplifies relative changes in EBIT into larger relative changes into larger relative changes in ROE and EPS. Operating leverage amplifies

a) Relative changes in EBIT into larger relative changes in sales revenue.

b) Relative changes in sales revenue into larger relative changes in EBIT

c) Relative changes in sales revenue relative changes in sales revenue into larger relative changes in ROE and EPS

d) Relative changes in ROE and EPS into larger relative changes in EBIT

418) Which one of the following methods serve to measure co relation between two variables?

a) Scatter diagram

b) Frequency distribution

c) Two-way table

d) Coefficient of Rank Corelation

419) Financial leverage is 2:1, Interest charges= Rs 20 L, Tax Rate=50%, Variable cost as % is 60 %, Fixed cost will be

a) Rs 1,20,00,000

b) Rs 40,00,000

c) Rs 80,00,000

d) Rs 1,80,00,000

420) Quiz in analog mass communication stories is

a) Static

b) Dynamic

c) I nteractive

d) Exploratory

421) Time value of money supports the comparison of cash flows recorded at different time period by

a) Discounting all cash flows at common point of time

b) Compounding all cash flows at common point of time

c) Using either a or b

d) None of the above

422) Attitudes, concepts, skills and knowledge are product of

a) Learning

b) Research

c) Heredity

d) Explanation

423) The value of plant and equipment worn out in the process of manufacturing goods and services is measured by

a) Intermediate production

b) Net National Product

c) Investment

d) Depreciation

e) Consumption

424) The statement containing various ledger balances on a particular date is called as

a) Trail balance

b) Balance sheet

c) Cash flow statement

d) None of these

425) Breakdown in verbal communication is called

a) Short circuit

b) Contradiction

c) Unevenness

d) Entropy

426) A motor car purchased for Rs 80,000 whose book value is Rs 48,000 was sold for Rs 1,00,000. Capital profit is

a) Rs 15,000

b) Rs 20,000

c) Rs 30,000

d) Rs 40,000

427) The communicated knowledge in a classroom is considered as

a) Non pervasive treasure

b) Limited judgement

c) Autonomous virtue

d) Cultural capital

428) Which of the following is true about financial statements?

a) Financial statements give a summary of accounts

b) Financial statements can be stated as recorded facts

c) Both A and B

d) None of the above

429) P is the father of R and S is the son of Q and T is the brother of P. If R is the sister of S, how is Q related to T.

a) Wife

b) Sister-in-Law

c) Brother-in-Law

d) Daughter in Law

430) Re-ordering level = Maximum consumption X

a) Minimum consumption

b) Maximum reorder period

c) Minimum reorder period

d) Both a and b

e) None of these

431) The teacher has been glorified by the phrase "Friend, philosopher and Guide because

a) He has to play all vital roles in the context of society

b) He transmits the high value of humanity to students

c) He is the great reformer of the society

d) He is a great patriot

432) COGS: Rs 50,000, GP Margin- 25 % of sales. Find out the value of sales

a) 2,00,000

b) 66,667

c) 66,500

d) None of these

433) In which of these activities, potential for nurturing creative and critical thinking is relatively greater?

a) Preparing a research summary

b) Presenting a seminar paper

c) Participation in research conference

d) Participation in workshop

434) Choose the correct order of components

1) Observation

2) Hypothesis making

3) Developing concepts

4) Deducing the consequences of theories

5) Methods employed to obtain them

1) 5,4,3,2,1

2) 1,3,2,4,5

3) 2,3,1,4,5

4) 4,5,3,2,1

435) Fixed Cost Rs 60,000 per annum, Product selling price Rs 20/Unit, Contribution to sales Ratio 40 %, Break Even Points in Units

a) 3000 units

b) 5000 units

c) 7500 units

d) 8000 units

436) Standard costing is the preparation of standard costs and their comparison with _____ and the analysis of ______

a) Marginal costs and variances

b) Variances, Marginal costs

b) Actual costs, Variances

a) Variances and Actual costs

437) Which of the following is an example of a maximum performance test?

a) Personality tests

b) Projective Personality tests

c) Aptitude tests

d) Interest and attitude scales

438) Opportunities to achieve further growth within current businesses are

a) Intensive opportunities

b) Integrative opportunities

c) Diversification opportunities

d) None of the above

439) Which of the following statements related to Contribution analysis are true?

a) If contribution is equal to zero, there is loss equal to fixed costs

b) If contribution is negative, loss is less than fixed costs

c) If contribution is positive and more than fixed costs there would be profit

d) All of the above

440) According to the CAPM (Capital Asset Pricing Model), a well-diversified portfolio's rate of return is a function of

a) Market risk

b) Unsystematic risk

c) Unique risk

d) Reinvestment risk

e) None of the above

441) Which of the following is not an argument?

a) Devadutt does not eat in the day so he must be eating at night

b) If Devadutt is growing fat and if he does not eat during the day, he will be eating at night

c) Devadutt eats in the night so he does not eat during the day

d) Since Devadutt does not eat in the day, he must be eating in the night

442) The spot price of an asset that pays no dividend is \$ 30 and the risk free rate for all maturities (with continuous compounding) is 10 % per annum. What is the three years forward price?

a) \$ 40

b) \$ 40.497

c) Rs 40.497

d) \$ 30

443) A computer has main memory of 960 Mbytes. What is the exact number of bytes contained in this memory?

a) 960×8

b) $960 \times 1024 \times 1024$

c) 960×1000

d) 960×1024

444) The teacher's role at the higher educational level is to

a) Provide information to students

b) Promote self-learning in students

c) Encourage healthy completion among students

d) Help students to solve their personal problem

445) Which among the following is best advantage of choice-based credit system?

a) Shift in focus from teacher-centric to student centric education

b) Improving classroom attendance

c) Helping teacher to complete syllabus on time

d) Reducing examination anxiety among students

446) During trade recession the goods are sold at

a) Depression price

b) Normal price

c) Minimum price

d) None of the above

447) Determine B.E.P in units and amount if units produced is Rs 10,000. Fixed cost is Rs 40,000. Selling price is Rs 50 per unit and variable cost is Rs 30 per unit

a) Rs 40 per unit, Rs 2,00,000

b) Rs 50 per unit, Rs 10,00,000

c) Rs 20 per unit, Rs 1,00,000

d) None of the above

448) All republics are grateful is taken true then which proposition is false

a) Republics are not grateful

b) Some republics are not grateful

c) No republics are grateful

d) Some republics are grateful

1) i

2) ii

3) i, ii, iii

4) ii, iii

449) Share capital of A Ltd is 20 L (2013),26 L (2014). Company asset of another company Rs 6 lac payable in fully paid shares incl - Goodwill (2L), Machinery (1.836L), Stock(2.164L). Fund from issue of shares

a) Rs 2,15,600

b) Rs 2,16,400

c) Rs 2,00,000

d) None of the above

450) The term current asset doesn't cover

a) Car

b) Debtors

c) Stock

d) Prepaid expenses

451) The term current asset includes -

a) Car

b) Accounts Receivables from Debtors

c) Stock

d) Prepaid expenses

452) The conceptual framework in which research is conducted is called as

a) Synopsis of research

b) Research design

c) Research hypothesis

d) Research paradigm

453) Media that exist in an inter-connected series of communication - points are referred to as:

a) Networked media

b) Connective media

c) Nodal media

d) Multimedia

454) If sales returns are Rs 25,000 sales are Rs 1,25,000 net purchases are Rs 84,000 and gross profit is Rs 21,000 then the cost of goods sold will be

a) Rs 84,000

b) Rs 64,000

c) Rs 79,000

d) Rs 92,000

455) Research has shown that the most frequent symptom of nervous instability among teachers is

a) Digestive upsets

b) Explosive behaviour

c) Fatigue

d) Worry

456) Which among the following statements are false?

A) When all figures in balance sheet are stated as percentage of total horizontal analysis

B) When all financial statements of several years are analysed - vertical analysis

C) Vertical analysis is also termed as dynamic analysis

a) Both A and B

b) Both A and C

c) Both B and C

d) A, B, C

457) A company that sells products to customer without demanding immediate payment but record it in balance sheet as

a) Account payable

b) Account receivable

c) Account equivalent

d) Account investment

458) When the bill is dishonoured, the account debited in the book of drawee

a) Acceptor's account

b) Creditors account

c) Bills payable account

d) None of the above

459) The major characteristic of corelation analysis is to seek out

a) Difference among variables

b) Variations among variables

c) Association among variables

d) Regression among variables

460) The major characteristic of co relation analysis is to seek out

a) Differences among variables

b) Variations among variables

c) Association among variables

d) Regression among variables

461) Translation loss may occur when

a) Exposed assets exceed exposed liabilities and foreign currency appreciates

b) Exposed assets exceed exposed liabilities and foreign currency depreciates

c) The subsidiary's balance sheet shows a loss

d) The foreign currency depreciates

462) Which of the following changes would constitute valid accounting transactions?

a) An increase in liability, increase in an asset

b) Increase in an asset decrease in proprietorship

c) Increase in a liability, decrease in an asset

d) All of the above

463) When a security or debt issue is under subscribed it is known as

a) Under subscription
b) High NET worth Individuals
c) Devolvement
d) All of the above

464) Which one of the following represents the binary equivalent of the decimal number 25"

a) 11011
b) 10101
c) 01101
d) 11001

465) Which of the following variables cannot be expressed in quantitative terms

a) Socio- economic status
b) Marital status
c) Numerical Aptitude
d) Professional attitude

466) ---- is generally a person who for consideration became possessor of a promissory note, bill of exchange or cheque'

a) Drawer in due course
b) Drawee in due course
c) Pawnor in due course
d) Pawnee in due course
e) Holder in due course

467) Action research is

a) Applied Research
b) Research carried out to solve immediate problems
c) Longitudinal research
d) All of the above

468) GST is a consumption of goods and service tax based on

a) Development
b) Dividend
c) Destiny
d) Duration
e) Destination

469) According to Swami Vivekanand's teachers' success depends on

a) His renunciation of personal gain and service to other's
b) His professional training and creativity
c) His concentration on his work and duties with a spirit of obedience to God
d) His mastery on the subject and capacity in controlling the students.

470) A global as opposed to international strategy involves

a) A wide variety of business strategies across countries
b) A single strategy for a subsidiary of a multinational firm
c) A single strategy for the entire global network of subsidiaries and partners
d) A wide variety of subsidiary strategies within the global network of subsidiaries

471) Converting a public company into a private company requires a special resolution

a) Passed by the members and with sanction of the central government
b) Passed by the members and approved by the Registrar of companies
c) Passed by the members and approved by the Company Law Tribunal
d) Passed by the members and approved by the auditors

472) One morning Udai and Vishal were talking to each other face to face at a crossing. If Vishal's shadow was exactly to the left of Udai, which direction was Udai facing

a) East

b) West

c) North

d) South

473) The transaction cost of trading of financial instruments in centralized market is classified as

a) Flexible costs

b) Low transaction costs

c) High transaction costs

d) Constant costs

474) The stock which has higher corelation with markets tend to have

a) High beta, less risky

b) Low beta, more risky

c) High beta, more risky

d) Low beta, less risky

475) In a certain coding method, the word QUESTION is encoded as DOMESTIC. In this coding, what is the code word for the word RESPONSE?

a) OMESUCEM

b) OMESICSM

c) OMESICEM

d) OMESISCM

476) According to the Black Scholes model, the purchaser can borrow fraction of security at risk free interest rate which is

a) Short term

b) Long term

c) Transaction cost

d) No transaction cost

477) Three partners A, B, C start a business. B's capital is 4 times C's capital and twice A's capital is equal to thrice B's capital. If the total profit is Rs 16,500 at the end of the year, find out B's share in it.

a) Rs 4000

b) Rs 5000

c) Rs 6000

d) Rs 7000

478) P is the father of R and S is the son of Q and T is the brother of P. If R is the sister of S, how is Q related to T.

a) Wife

b) Sister -in-law

c) Brother in-law

d) Daughter in law

479) In circulation of net cash flow, the depreciation and amortization are treated as

a) Current liabilities

b) Income expenses

c) Non-cash revenues

d) Non-cash charges

480) If holder of a bill of exchange allows drawee more than ---- hours, exclusive of public holidays to consider whether he will accept all previous parties not consenting to such allowances are thereby discharged from liability to such holder

a) 24

b) 12

c) 36?

d) 48

e) 60

481) Which of the following skills are needed for present day teacher to adjust effectively with classroom teaching?

a) Knowledge of technology

b) Use of technology in teaching learning

c) Knowledge of student's needs

d) Content mastery

a) 1 & 3

b) 2 & 3

c) 2,3 & 4

d) 2 & 4

482) A technique of lowering the risk for multinational companies and globally designed portfolios is classified as

a) National diversification

b) Behavioural diversification

c) Gobal diversification

d) Behavioural finance

483) Premium received on issue of shares cannot be utilized for

a) Distribution of question

b) For the issue of bonus shares

c) For writing of preliminary expenses

d) For providing premium payable on redemption

484) Which of the following is not the critical feature of qualitative research?

a) Actual settings are the direct source of data

b) Data takes the form of words or pictures

c) Seeking to establish relationships among measured social facts

d) Researchers becomes immersed in the situation, present or past related to the phenomenon

485) Assertion: All teaching should aim at ensuring learning.

Reason: All learning results from teaching

1) Both (A) AND ® are true and R is the correct explanation of (A)

2) Both (A) AND ® are true but R is not the correct explanation of (A)

3) (A) is true but ® is false

4) (A) is false but ® is true

486) In a statement of cash flows, a company investing in short term financial investments and in fixed assets results in

a) Increased cash

b) Decreased cash

c) Increased liabilities

d) Increased equity

487) Transaction by which A promised to pay B and C for consideration during their joint lives and after death of one of them, to survivor, the consideration moved from B but the agreements were signed by all three i.e. A, B, & C

a) There was privity between A and B but not with C

b) There was privity between A and C but not with B

c) There was privity between A on one side and C on the other side

d) None of these

488) If the proposition "All men are not true" is true then which inference is correct.

1) All men are mortal is true

2) Some men are mortal is false

3) No men are mortal is doubtful

4) All men are mortal

a) 1,2,3

b) 2,3,4

c) 1,3,4

d) 1 and 3

489) The negative minimum risk portfolio of any security shows that market security sold

a) Less than original price

b) Greater than original price

c) Equal to original price

d) Equal to sum of stocks

490) Which of the following statement is not correct about GST?

a) GST is like a last point retail tax. GST is going to be collected at the point of sale.

b) GST will abolish all the direct tax levied in India

c) It will be implemented from 1st July 2017 throughout the country

d) It will unify the tax structure

491) A researcher uses parametric test in lieu of non-parametric test for analysis and interpretation of results. This may be described as a case of

a) Unethical research practice

b) Malpractice in reporting of results

c) Technical lapse in handling data

d) Manipulation of research results

492) SGST is applicable when

a) Goods are sold within a state

b) Goods are sold from one GST dealer to a customer

c) Goods are sold by a GST dealer to another GST dealer

d) Interstate supply

493) A current account trade deficit means that

a) Spending on imported goods and services equals the export earnings over a given period

b) Spending on imported goods and services is greater than the export earnings over a given period

c) Spending on imported goods and services is less than the export earnings over a given period

d) Government spending on imported goods and services equals the export earnings over a given period

494) Identify questions, which are called processes rather than content based questions:

1) Convergent questions

2) Divergent questions

3) Fact based questions

4) Concept based questions

5) Open questions

6) Closed questions

a) 1,2,3

b) 2,3,4

c) 4,5,6

d) 2,3,5

495) In applying Vogel's approximation method to a profit maximization problem, row and column penalties are determined by

a) Finding the largest unit cost in each row or column

b) Finding the smallest unit cost in each row or column

c) Finding the difference between the two lowest unit costs in each row and column

d) Finding the difference between the two highest unit costs in each row and column

496) Reconciliation statement under Form 9 c shall be done after the preparation of

a) Audited financial statement

b) Annual return of GST

c) Tax audit

d) Both a and b

497) Identify non probability sampling procedures

a) Simple random sampling

b) Dimensional sampling

c) Snowball sampling

d) Cluster sampling

e) Quota sampling

f) Stratified sampling

1) i, ii, iii

2) ii, iv, v

3) i, iii, v

4) ii, iii, v

498) Artifacts that arise and affect the internal validity in research are

a) History

b) Randomization

c) Maturity

d) Instrumentation

e) Experimental mortality

f) Matching

1) a, b, c, d

2) b, c, d, f

3) a, c, d, e

4) d, e, f, b

499) A profit maximizing perfect competitor is in short run equilibrium with an output of 100 per day. Which of the following events would not cause it to alter its output in the short-run?

a) A change in the demand for the product it makes

b) A change in the number of other firms in its industry

c) A change in the price of a fixed output

d) A change in the price of a variable input

500) A special audit under GST is conducted by

a) Commissioner

b) CGST official

c) CAG

d) CA/CMA

Answer Key Mock Test - 5

401) b) False
402) c) Both I and II are implied
403) b) Problem formulation and reporting of research findings
404) d) SEIN CPAMO
405) a) Current assets-stock-Prepaid expenses
406) c) Increase in trade receivables
407) a) Both (A) & (R) are true and (R) is the correct explanation of A
408) a) MM proposition I with no tax
409) b) STRIDE
410) b) Positive as equity holders gain the tax shield on the debt interest
411) a) Market Price per share /Earnings per share
412) 3) a, b, c, f
413) b) Maximises the value of the firm
414) c) Address the issue of global climate change
415) a) Interest tax shield
416) b) Military purposes
417) b) Relative changes in sales revenue into larger relative changes in EBIT
418) d) Coefficient of Rank Corelation
419) c) Rs 80,00,000
420) a) Static
421) c) Using either a or b
422) a) Learning
423) d) Depreciation
424) a) Trail balance
425) d) Entropy
426) b) Rs 20,000
427) d) Cultural capital
428) c) Both A and B
429) b) Sister-in-Law
430) b) Maximum reorder period
431) b) He transmits the high value of humanity to students
432) b) 66,667
433) c) Participation in research conference
434) 2) 1,3,2,4,5
435) c) 7500 units
436) c) Actual costs, Variances
437) c) Aptitude tests
438) a) Intensive opportunities
439) a) If contribution is equal to zero, there is loss equal to fixed costs
440) a) Market risk
441) b) If Devadutt is growing fat and if he does not eat during the day, he will be eating at night
442) b) $40.497
443) b) 960 × 1024 × 1024
444) b) Promote self-learning in students
445) a) Shift in focus from teacher-centric to student centric education
446) a) Depression price
447) c) Rs 20 per unit, Rs 1,00,000
448) 3) i, ii, iii
449) b) Rs 2,16,400
450) a) Car
451) b) Accounts Receivables from Debtors
452) b) Research design
453) a) Networked media
454) c) Rs 79,000
455) b) Explosive behaviour
456) b) Both A and C
457) b) Account receivable
458) c) Bills payable account
459) c) Association among variables
460) c) Association among variables
461) b) Exposed assets exceed exposed liabilities and foreign currency depreciates
462) a) An increase in liability, increase in an asset
463) c) Devolvement
464) d) 11001
465) d) Professional attitude
466) e) Holder in due course
467) b) Research carried out to solve immediate problems
468) e) Destination
469) a) His renunciation of personal gain and service to other's

470) c) A single strategy for the entire global network of subsidiaries and partners
471) a) Passed by the members and with sanction of the central government
472) c) North
473) b) Low transaction costs
474) c) High beta, more risky
475) c) OMESICEM
476) a) Short term
477) c) Rs 6000
478) b) Sister -in-law
479) d) Non-cash charges
480) d) 48
481) c) 2, 3 & 4
482) c) Global diversification
483) a) Distribution of question
484) c) Seeking to establish relationships among measured social facts
485) 3) (A) is true but ® is false
486) b) Decreased cash
487) c) There was privity between A on one side and C on the other side
488) b) 2,3,4
489) a) Less than original price
490) b) GST will abolish all the direct tax levied in India
491) c) Technical lapse in handling data
492) a) Goods are sold within a state
493) b) Spending on imported goods and services is greater than the export earnings over a given period
494) d) 2,3,5
495) d) Finding the difference between the two highest unit costs in each row and column
496) d) Both a and b
497) 4) ii, iii, v
498) 3) a, c, d, e
499) c) A change in the price of a fixed output
500) d) CA/CMA

Practice Mock Test - 6

501) A shift in attitude in respondents between two points during data collection is called

a) Reactive effect

b) Maturation effect

c) Regression effect

d) Conditioning effect

502) Which of the following statements about the market supply curve for a product is false?

a) Market supply curves represent individual supply curves of all firms producing product added together

b) Market supply curves may shift if there is change in behaviour of some firms which produce product

c) Market supply curves may shift if there is change in the price of the product

d) Market supply curves may shift if there is change in the number of firms which supply the product

503) In which of the following cases, Advance ruling under GST cannot be sought?

a) Determination of time and value of supply of goods or services or both

b) Determination of whether a particular transaction is supply of goods or services or both.

c) Applicability of a notification issued under CGST act

504) Didactic communication is

a) Intra personal

b) Inter personal

c) Organizational;

d) Relational

505) The ratio between cash in hand and total assets maintained by the banks is called

a) SBR (Statutory Bank Ratio)

b) SLR (Statutory Liquid Ratio)

c) CBR (Central Bank Reserve)

d) CLR (Central Liquid Reserve)

506) A null hypothesis is

a) When there is no difference between the variables

b) The same as research hypothesis

c) Subjective in nature

d) When there is difference between the variables

507) What is most likely to increase in a monopoly market compared to a competitive market?

a) Consumer surplus is likely to increase

b) Consumer surplus is likely to decrease

c) Producer surplus is likely to increase

d) Social welfare is likely to increase

508) If a minor draw, endorse, deliver and negotiates Negotiable instruments it binds

a) All the parties except minor
b) All the parties including minor
c) Minor only
d) Minor and the Drawee

509) The factors which are most important in determining the impact of anthropogenic activities on environment are

a) Population, forest cover and land available per person
b) Population, affluence per person and land available per person
c) Population, affluence per person and the technology used for exploiting resources
d) Atmospheric conditions, population and forest cover

510) Biomagnification means increase in the

a) Concentration of pollutants in living organisms
b) Number of species
c) Size of living organisms
d) Biomass

511) In game theory when a business chooses the best of the worst outcomes this is called

a) A mini- mini strategy
b) A mini-sum
c) A maxi-maxi strategy
d) A maxi-min strategy

512) Which of the following service is taxable under RCM in the hands of recipient of said service?

a) Transportation of goods by a GTA to unregistered person
b) Legal services provided by an Advocate to an NGO registered under GST
c) Renting of shops by municipality to a registered person
d) Security services provided by an unregistered entity to registered business entity

513) Deductive reasoning proceeds from

a) One general conclusion to another general conclusion
b) General to particular
c) One particular conclusion to another particular conclusion
d) Particular to general

514) Which of the following is taxable supply under GST Act>

a) Transportation of deceased person through a hired vehicle
b) Gift of office laptop by an employer to its employee on which ITC availed
c) A new laptop worth Rs 45,000 by an employer to its employee
d) Fines/penalty/LD paid by a contractor to government for delay/ non-performance of contract
e) Gift of merchandise goods given by a registered person to its customers

515) Good evaluation of written material should not be based on

a) Linguistic expression
b) Logistic presentation
c) Ability to reproduce whatever is read
d) Comprehension of subject

516) Local content ratios mean that a minimum percentage of a product must consist of locally produced or sourced components

a) True, b) False

517) M/s crafty, Rajasthan un-registered handicraft dealer. Self-transport to Delhi 45,000 Handicrafts. Tax of

Intercepted, asked for E way Bill. Driver- E Way Bill not required. Value of consignment less than 50,000

a) E-way bill is required in case of interstate supply, only if value supply is mor than Rs 50,000

b) E-way bill is required in case of taxable goods

c) E-way bill is not required when supplied by an unregistered person

d) E-way is mandatory for interstate supply of Handicraft goods irrespective of value of consignment.

518) The term phenomenology is associated with the process of

a) Qualitative Research

b) Analysis of Variance

c) Co-relational study

d) Probability sampling

519) A surety is discharged if the creditor, without consent, unconditionally releases the principal- debtor, the reason for this principle being that:

a) The release extinguishes the principal obligation

b) Such release adversely affects the right of surety to sue principal-debtor.

c) Deprives surety his right to compel debtor to perform his own obligation to the creditor.

d) a, b & c

520) Which one of the following is the process of entrepreneurs developing new products that overtime make current products obsolete?

a) New Business Model

b) Anatomization

c) Creative destruction

d) None of the above given options

521) Generalized conclusion on the basis of a sample is technically known as

a) Data analysis and interpretation

b) Parameter inference

c) Statistical inference

d) All of the above

522) The Diamond model assumes that

a) Multinational firms must develop global strategies based only on home demand conditions.

b) Multinational firms must pay less attention to global consumers than domestic consumers

c) The national home base of a firm must be the biggest market fo a multinational firm.

d) National home base of a firm plays key rle in shaping firm's competitive advantage in global markets

523) Which code is used to classify goods and services under GST?

a) HSN code

b) SAC/HSN Code

c) GST Code

d) SAC Code

524) Which of the following s not a critical feature of qualitative research?

a) Actual settings are the direct sources of data.

b) Data takes the form of words or pictures

c) Seeking to establish relationship among measured social facts

d) Researcher becomes immersed in the situation, resent or past related to the phenomenon

525) The main advantage of deemed prospectus is that the companycan save underwriting expenses

a) Shelf prospectus

b) Red Herring prospectus

c) Abridged prospectus

d) Deemed prospectus

526) The factors which are most important in determining the impact of anthropogenic activities on environment are

a) Population, forest cover and land available per person

b) Population, affluence per person and land available per person

c) Population, affluence per person and the technology used for exploring resources

d) Atmospheric conditions, population and forest cover

527) Suppose a profit making unregulated natural monopoly is brought under the control of regulator who requires it in future to follow a marginal cost pricing rule

a) The monopoly would move from making a profit to making a loss.

b) The monopoly would reduce its output

c) The monopoly would now set its output where its MC curve intersects its AR curve

d) The monopolists' price would now equal its marginal cost

528) Find the wrong number in the sequence: 125, 127,130,135,142, 153,165

a) 130

b) 142

c) 153

d) 165

529) In which of these problems is the actual message lost in the abundance of transmitted information

a) Selecting perception

b) Over communication

c) Under communication

d) Filtering

530) The Porter Diamond Model suggests that four factors determine a firm's competitive advantage

1) Home demand conditions, home supply conditions, firm strategy and structure, supporting industries

2) Home demand and factors, firm strategy and rivalry related industry, supporting industry

3) Home demand condition, home factor condition, firm structure & rivalry

4) Home demand conditions, home supply, firm strategy, related and supporting industries

531) PEST analysis is

a) A broad framework to help managers understand the environment in which their business operates

b) A checklist to ask how political, economic strategic or technological developments can influence

c) A checklist for forecasting political, economic, strategic or technological factors

d) A framework for strategic analysis of internal and external environment

532) An optimal business partner in a successful international strategic alliance should have 2 key qualities

a) Corporate culture fit and national culture fit

b) Partner related criterion and task related criterion

c) Cultural fit and trust

d) Strategic fit and cultural fit

533) Internalization stimuli refer to (Internal/External)

a) Internal motives for foreign investment

b) Internal factors arising within organization- influence a firm's decision to develop & sustain

c) A multinational's firm's motives for establishing an investment in a foreign location

d) Factors influencing a firm's decision to initiate, develop, sustain in business activities

534) Which of the following is not one of the qualities which makes debt attractive to firms?

a) Cost of debt is generally less than cost of share capital, can lower overall cost of capital for firm

b) Debt interest only gets paid when the company is making a profit

c) It reduces the amount of corporate tax payable by firms by reducing the amount of taxable profit

d) Required return on debt is lower from lender's point of view, debt is less risky than equity

535) By definition, currency appreciation occurs when

a) The value of all currencies fail relative to gold

b) The value of all currencies rise relative to gold

c) The value of one currency rises relative to another currency

d) The value of one currency falls relative to another currency

536) Goal 17 is bout strengthening the means of implementation and revitalizing the "Global Partnership" for realizing all the other Goals. Which of the following is not part of Goal 17?

a) Mobilizing the financial resources necessary to achieve the goals.

b) Creating international sports tournaments and festivals to promote the goals

c) Helping developing countries build the capacities needed in areas, technology, public policy

d) Enhancing trade, especially to help developing countries increase exports and grow their economies

537) Which of the following is typically the most important economy or synergy which is sought from Mergers and Acquisitions M&A activity?

a) Economics of scope from applying existing resources to new uses, at little additional cost.

b) Revenue and marketing synergies from new, enhanced or more efficient distribution

c) Economics of scale effects from organizational learning

d) Economics of scale from doing away with duplication of function between the two firms

538) If the cross elasticity of demand is 2

a) The products are substitutes and demand is cross price elastic

b) The products are substitutes and demand is cross price inelastic

c) The products are complements and demand is cross price elastic

d) The products are complements and demand is cross price

539) Which of the following is not a limitation of ratio analysis?

a) Differences in accounting policies may detract from value of inter-firm companies

b) Ratios do not provide explanations for changes found

c) Fin statements and accounting ratios can be distorted by as a result of "one off large transactions.

d) Ratios highlight underlying trends

540) A table with all possible value of a random variable and its corresponding probabilities is called

a) Probability mass function

b) Probability density function

c) Cumulative distribution function

d) Probability distribution

541) Normal distribution is applied for

a) Continuous random distribution

b) Discrete random variable

c) Irregular random variable

d) Uncertain random variable

542) For which of the following distributions mean and variance are equal?

a) Normal distribution

b) Poisson distribution

c) Binomial distribution

d) Negative binomial distribution

543) The modern theory of the firm hold that firms behave in a way that is designed to maximize

a) Profit

b) Value of the firm

c) Total revenue

d) Monopoly power

544) What advantage do objective types tests have over essay type tests?

a) Easier to interpret

b) Regularly require less technical knowledge

c) The sampling content can be wider

d) They take less time to prepare

545) When the price of the underlying asset increases then the good option is

a) Buy the call option

b) Sell the call option

c) Buy the put option

d) Sell the put option

546) Consider the buying of put option, the probability that the buyer would have negative payoff increases with the

a) Increase in stock price

b) Decrease in stock price

c) Increase in maturity duration

d) Decrease in maturity duration

547) In primary markets, the property of shares which made it easy to sell newly issued security is considered as

a) Increased liquidity

b) Decreased liquidity

c) Money flow

d) Large funds

548) According to Maslow's Hierarchy of Needs theory, the need for fulfilment, for realizing one's own potential and for fully using one's talents and capabilities are example of ---- needs

a) Self-actualization

b) Physiological

c) Social

d) Esteem

549) Which of the following is not a result of recognizing the importance of ethnic groups by marketers?

a) Use of an undifferentiated one-size-fits all marketing strategy

b) Different pricing strategies for different groups

c) Variations in product offerings to suit the wants of a particular group

d) Study of ethnic buying habits to isolate market segments

550) The nominal interest rates and the nominal cash flows usually reflect the

a) Inflation effects

b) Opportunity effects

c) Equity effects

d) Debt effects

551) Discretionary behaviour that is not part of an employee's formal job requirements, but that promotes the effective functioning of the organization;

a) Behaviour

b) Organizational Behaviour

c) Workplace Behaviour

d) Organizational citizenship Behaviour

552) The companies take savings as premiums, invest in bonds and make payment to beneficiaries are classified as:

a) Debit unions

b) Life insurance companies

c) Credit unions

d) Auto purchases

553) In Baumol's model, the size of the profit constraint faced by an individual firm is likely to be relatively high in all the below cases with the exception of when:

a) Profits made by rival firms are increasing

b) The number of shareholders increase as major current shareholders rekease their shares

c) The overall state of the market is buoyant

d) Profits declared by the firm in previous time high periods were high

554) In a statement of cash flows a company investing in short term financial investments and in fixed assets results in

a) Increased cash

b) Decreased cash

c) Increased liabilities

d) Increased equity

555) In put call parity relationship, the put option minus call option in addition with stock is equal to

a) Exercise price present value

b) Exercise price future value

c) Time line value

d) Time value of bond

556) The balanced scorecard perspective measures company's success in targeted segments of customers, this perspective can also be classified as

a) Internal business process perspective

b) Customer perspective

c) Learning perspective

d) Financial perspective

557) Which of the following processes is not fundamental in explaining how consumers think and learn about products and brands?

a) Cognition

b) Perception

c) Learning

d) Personality

558) Any statement whose validity is tested on the basis of a sample is called

a) Null hypothesis

b) Alternative hypothesis

c) Statistical hypothesis

d) Simple hypothesis

559) A quantitative statement about a population is called

a) Research hypothesis

b) Composite hypothesis

c) Simple hypothesis

d) Statistical hypothesis

560) Which of the following correctly lists computer memory types from highest to lowest speed?

a) Secondary storage, Main memory (RAM), Cache memory, CPU Registers

b) CPU Registers, Cache memory, Secondary storage, Main memory (RAM),

c) CPU Registers, Cache memory, Main memory (RAM), Secondary storage

d) Cache memory, CPU Registers, Main memory (RAM), Secondary storage

561) Which of the following is a characteristic of Web 2.0 Applications?

a) Multiple users schedule their time to use Web 2.0 Applications one by one.

b) Web 2.0 Applications are focussed on the ability for people to collaborate and share information online

c) Web 2.0 Applications provide users with content rather than facilitating uses to create it.

d) Web 2.0 Applications use only static pages.

562) When employee(s) are coming to work daily and be available for job, but are less productive than usual and as expected from.?

a) Quite Vacationing

b) Quite Quitting

c) Coffee Badging

d) Baby Boomers

e) Moonlighting

563) An organization if sells goods, without receiving its sales price upfront, then such amount is referred as trade payables.

564) Credit sales time period should be less than payables time period.

565) Inventory outstanding days should be less than total days for trade receivables.

566) A moderate policy of firm towards working capital, suggests that it neither more nor less of cash at hand / cash at bank.

567) An aggressive cash management policy of firm is when it has idle cash at hand / cash at bank available.

568) The balance sheet concept of working capital focuses upon matching current asset to current liabilities and/or having surplus current asset over current liabilities.

569) The Operating cycle concept of working capital focuses upon receipts and disbursements raw material and finished goods.

570) Identify correct formula:

a) [Average inventory ÷ Cost of sales] * 365 = Inventory conversion period

b) Average inventory × [Cost of sales ÷ 365] = Inventory conversion period

c) Average inventory + [Cost of sales ÷ 365] = Inventory conversion period

d) Average inventory = [Cost of sales ÷ 365] ÷ Inventory conversion period

571) STATEMENT 1: If average inventory is Rs. 42000 with cost of sales at Rs. 17000. Then the inventory conversion period is for 1901.86 days.

STATEMENT 2: The conservation policy of working capital focuses on larger current ratio, with more of cash at hand /bank.

a) Both statement are correct.

b) Statement 1 is correct and statement 2 is incorrect.

c) Statement 1 is incorrect and statement 2 is correct.

d) Both statement are incorrect.

572) Identify correct formula:

a) Operating cycle + Payable Deferral Period = Cash conversion cycle

b) Operating cycle - Payable Deferral Period = Cash conversion cycle

c) Operating cycle × Payable Deferral Period = Cash conversion cycle

d) Operating cycle ÷ Payable Deferral Period = Cash conversion cycle

573) If trade payables of firm are Rs. 72000 with wages payable for Rs. 28000. The total cost of sales being Rs. 30000 with no other additional expenses, for the deferred period. The Payable Deferred Period is:

a) 33.3 days

b) 6.667 days

c) 3.3 days

d) 33 days

574) The firms total current assets are referred as Gross working capital.

575) Portion of current assets available readily for working capital use is net working capital such as:

5L (current assets) - 3L (current liabilities) = 2L (net working capital)

576) The greater the cost of sales compared to trade payables, the less will be the trade payables deferral period.

577) Vendor financing, also known as negative cash conversion cycle, where the manufacturer buys the raw material but sells goods on credit. (True)

578) Identify the correct formula:

a) CCC = DIO ÷ DSO × DPO

b) CCC = DIO + DSO - DPO

c) CCC = DIO - DSO + DPO

d) CCC = DIO + DSO × DPO

579) The firm has annual sales of Rs. 50 lakh, with accounts receivable of rs. 5,00,000. Calculate days of sales outstanding. (1 year = 365 days)

a) 37 days

b) 365 days

c) 42 days

d) 49 days

580) A firm has accounts payable for Rs. 13,00,000 and cost of goods sold were Rs. 30,00,000. Calculate days payables outstanding?

a) 167 days

b) 15 days

c) 19 days

d) 158 days

581) International transactions undergo foreign exchange risk exposure.

582) Translation risk is determined as risk exposure due to non-receipt of raw material from foreign location.

583) Transaction risk exposure occurs due to change in foreign currency exchanging rate at the time of entering the transaction and at the time of realizing the transaction.

584) Interest rate parity theory suggests that a parity in currency of two countries will result due to parity in interest rates of such countries.

585) An organization with foreign transactions which are exposed to foreign exchange risk) can buy currency futures, in a way to almost eliminate risk of loss occurring due to foreign exchange risks.

586) A risk off setting can be initiated if a firm buys currency swap simultaneously along with a foreign currency transaction, of same countries.

587) An organization with domestic bound receivables, enters into currency swap for gain purpose company is doing______

588) Transaction risk exposure due to domestic trade to domestic trade receivables, can be offsetted through netting (off) practice of firm, via a buy/sale of currency swap, etc.

589) Foreign market entry for sale of domestically produced goods is initiated after country risk analysis, as in, when there is no risk , is when a firm should enter such country.

590) Operating exposures are different from translation exposure.

591) Cross - border investments can be evaluated through cross - border capital budgeting.

592) The present value interest rates and discounting rates are similar (PV table) for two countries.

593) Present value interest rates are governed through central banks of countries.

594) Floating rate of interest based loans if issued in the country more, such countries 'currency swap if bought shall witness ups and downs' in terms of losses / gains on swaps.

595) An organisation has days payables outstanding as 58 and days of sales outstanding as 132 and had a cash conversion cycle of 179. Calculate days of inventory outstanding.

a) 79

b) 74

c) 105

d) None

596) A firm has a accounts receivable of Rs.25000/- and total credit sales made were of Rs.134000/- for a period of 364 days. The days of sales outstanding are:

a) 91 days

b) 84 days

c) 16 days

d) 68 days

597) A firm has accounts payable of Rs.74000/- with COGS of Rs.2.98 Lac for a period of 364 days. Calculate days payable outstanding:

a) 90 days

b) 97 days

c) 118 days

d) 78 days

598) **XYZ Ltd. Had set Maximum cash position as Rs.15000 and return point of Rs.7000/-. The receivables of Rs.34000/- were realised and the firm sold its investment then. According to Miller-Orr Cash Management was done:**

a) Correct

b) Incorrect

599) **XYZ Ltd. Had set Maximum cash position as Rs.15000 and return point of Rs.7000/-. The receivables of Rs.34000/- were realised and the firm made an investment of Rs.27000/- then. According to Miller-Orr, Cash Management was done:**

a) Correct

b) Incorrect

600) **An organisation has cash flow requirement of Rs.20000/-, where its interest rate is 4% and transaction cost was 15%. Calculate the cash spread and return point of cash position:**

a) 62000, 19000

b) 78562, 18562

c) 55688, 18563

d) None of the above

Answer Key Mock Test - 6

501) c) regression effect
502) c) Market supply curves may shift if there is change in the price of the product
503) b) Determination of whether a particular transaction is supply of goods or services or both.
504) b) Inter personal
505) b) SLR (Statutory Liquid Ratio)
506) a) when there is no difference between the variables
507) c) Producer surplus is likely to increase
508) a) All the parties except minor
509) c) Population, affluence per person and the technology used for exploiting resources
510) a) concentration of pollutants in living organisms
511) d) A maxi-min strategy
512) c) Renting of shops by municipality to a registered person
513) Deductive reasoning proceeds from a) one general conclusion to another general conclusionb) general to particularc) one particular conclusion to another particular conclusiond) particular to general
514) b) Gift of office laptop by an employer to its employee on which ITC availed
515) d) Comprehension of subject
516) a) True
517) d) E way is mandatory for interstate supply of Handicraft goods irrespective of value of consignment.
518) a) Qualitative Research
519) d) a, b & c
520) c) Creative destruction
521) a) Data analysis and interpretation
522) d) National home base of a firm plays key rle in shaping firm's competitive advantage in global markets
523) b) SAC/HSN Code
524) c) Seeking to establish relationship among measured social facts
525) d) Deemed prospectus
526) c) population, affluence per person and the technology used for exploring resources
527) b) The monopoly would reduce its output
528) d) 165
529) b) Over communication
530) 3) home demand condition, home factor condition, firm structure & rivalry
531) a) a broad framework to help managers understand the environment in which their business operates
532) d) Strategic fit and cultural fit
533) d) factors influencing a firm's decision to initiate, develop, sustain in business activities
534) b) Debt interest only gets paid when the company is making a profit
535) c) the value of one currency rises relative to another currency
536) b) creating international sports tournaments and festivals to promote the goals
537) d) Economics of scale from doing away with duplication of function between the two firms
538) c) The products are complements and demand is cross price elastic
539) d) Ratios highlight underlying trends
540) d) Probability distribution
541) a) Continuous random distribution
542) b) Poisson distribution
543) b) Value of the firm
544) c) The sampling content can be wider
545) a) Buy the call option
546) a) increase in stock price
547) a) Increased liquidity
548) a) self-actualization
549) a) Use of an undifferentiated one-size-fits all marketing strategy
550) a) inflation effects
551) c) Workplace Behaviour
552) b) life insurance companies

553) b) The number of shareholders increase as major current shareholders rekease their shares
554) b) Decreased cash
555) In put call parity relationship, the put option minus call option in addition with stock is equal to a) exercise price present valueb) exercise price future valuec) time line valued) time value of bond
556) b) Customer perspective
557) d) Personality
558) c) Statistical hypothesis
559) d) Statistical hypothesis
560) c) CPU Registers, Cache memory, Main memory (RAM), Secondary storage
561) b) Web 2.0 Applications are focussed on the ability for people to collaborate and share information online
562) b) Quite Quitting
563) (False)
564) (True)
565) (True)
566) (True)
567) (False)
568) (True)
569) (True)
570) Ans-(A)
571) Ans-(C)
572) Ans-(B)
573). c) 3.3 days
574) (True)
575) (True)
576) (True)
577) (True)
578) b)
579) a) 37 days
580) Ans-(D)
581) True
582) False
583) True
584) False
585) True
586) False
587) Correct
588) False
589) False
590) True
591) True
592) False
593) True
594) False
595) C
596) D
597) A
598) Incorrect
599) Correct
600) C.

- Spread = 3[3/4(0.15*20000/0.04)] 1/3
- Spread = 55687.50
- Return Point = Spread/3 = 55687.50/3 = 18562.50.

Practice Mock Test - 7

1) Which of the following is necessary to understand banking rates of interest?

a) Financial Statement Analysis

b) Capital Budgeting

c) Time Value of Money

d) All of the above

2) A store advertises a product at a low price but doesn't intend to sell it, instead convincing customers to buy a more expensive model.

a) Insufficient stock

b) Bait and Switch

c) False Claims

d) Deceptive Advertising

3) Which of the following is the goal of HR towards their efficient employees?

a) Personnel workshop

b) Career Management

c) Career Plateau

d) All of the above

4) Making promises of promotion but never following through. Displaying a lack of interest in the employee's career progress is known as

a) Wallowing

b) Breadcrumbing

c) Ghosting

d) All of the above

5) Which of the following sells the product at maximum retail price?

a) Hyperstores

b) Dark stores

c) Mom and Pop Stores

d) All of the above

6) A feeling of workplace disengagement resulting into a type of leave from employer is known as

a) Casual Leave

b) Sick Leave

c) Mental Illness Leave

d) Unhappy Leave

7) Which act covers welfare measures for working women?

a) Maternity Benefits Act

b) Companies Act

c) Gratuity act

d) Factories Act

8) Which of the following concepts, essentially carry the Fundamental of Value Creation?

a) Product Concept

b) Selling Concept

c) Marketing Concept

d) Societal Marketing Concept

9) A store used by online Apps to hold and then disburse customer orders:

a) Hyperstore

b) Dark store

c) E-stores

d) E Commerce stores

10) STATEMENT I - Price gouging leads to stagflation, after demand shock period is over.

STATEMENT II - A sample of 400 male students is found to have a mean height of 67.47 inches. Can it be regarded as a sample from a large population with mean height 67.47 inches and standard deviation.

a) Both STATEMENTS are True

b) Both STATEMENTS are False

c) STATEMENT I is correct, STATEMENT II is incorrect.

d) STATEMENT I is incorrect, STATEMENT II is correct.

11) If there is partial employment in the country, and competitive exams are negative processes of selection, educational qualification is a yardstick to earn livelihood which is

a) Economics of Development

b) Economics of Application

c) Economics of Discrimination

d) Both A and B

12) When aggregate income increases, consumption expenditure also increases but

a) By a somewhat large amount.

b) By a somewhat small amount.

c) Both A and B

d) None of the above.

13) Bank submissions for overnight, 1/3/6/12 month <u>USD</u> settings will cease as of end June 2023 after which representative <u>LIBOR</u> rates will no longer be available.

a) USD

b) USD, LIBOR

c) INR

d) LIBOR

14) A firm in late growth phase, decides on unrelated diversification from current product line. It's future call derivative will be signed at

a) Exercise price more than strike price.

b) Exercise price less than strike price.

c) Exercise price same as strike price.

d) None of the above

15) A performance appraisal technique that makes use of feedback from supervisors, subordinates and co-workers is known as:

a) Work oriented appraisal

b) 360-degree feedback

c) Informal appraisal

d) Graphic rating

16) According to Hertzberg 2 Factor theory, which factors are not motivational factors?

a) Satisfaction

b) Hygiene factors

c) Salary

d) None of the above

17) ____ is a contract / financial instrument for an organization through which an employee when receives salary is supposed to payback a fixed % of their income.

a) Compensation package

b) CTC

c) International Solar Alliance

d) Income Sharing Agreement Correct answer: DExplanation- In order to help organizations save on their taxes they enter into certain arrangements with their employees wherein they pay a higher salary only to take back certain portion of it in cash showing as total salary of expenses and thereof helping organization reduce its tax liabilities.

18) **According to which doctrine axing the law, if in case, some particular provision of a statute offends or is against a constitutional limitation, but that provision is severable from the rest of the statute, only that offending**

a) Doctrine severability

b) Doctrine of eclipse

c) Doctrine of waiver

d) Doctrine of territorial news

19) **---- contains a list of central and state laws that cannot be challenged in court of law and was added by the constitution as the 1st amendment act, 1951, by the Govt of Pandit Nehru**

a) Schedule 12

b) Schedule 11

c) Schedule 9

d) Schedule 1

20) **Statement 1: Managers must develop healthy relations with various groups in order to achieve the goals smoothly.**

Statement 2: Managers work only with internal people (subordinates, supervisors, peers) and not with external people.

a) Both 1 and 2 are correct

b) Both 1 and 2 are incorrect

c) Statement 1 is correct and statement 2 is incorrect

d) Statement 1 is incorrect and statement 2 is correct

21) **For economic growth and meeting the demands of inflation, the RBI Act 1934 recommended constitution of a statutory body as per**

a) 4B(3C), RBI Act,1857

b) 45ZB, RBI Act, 1934

c) 45ZB, Constitutional Amendment Act, 1943

d) 54ZB, RBI Act,1938

22) **Statement 1: Managers play the figurehead role when they perform duties that are ceremonial and symbolic in nature.**

Statement 2: Receiving and communicating information are perhaps the most important aspects of a manager.

a) Both 1 and 2 are correct

b) Both 1 and 2 are incorrect

c) Statement 1 is correct and statement 2 is incorrect

d) Statement 1 is incorrect and statement 2 is correct

23) **Statement 1: An accounting manager supervises the accounting function**

Statement 2: The manager of production supervises engineers and support staff engaged in design of a product or service.

a) Both 1 and 2 are correct

b) Both 1 and 2 are incorrect

c) Statement 1 is correct and statement 2 is incorrect

d) Statement 1 is incorrect and statement 2 is correct

24) **Which of the following related to CSR theories is correct?**

a) Institutional theory is based on the shareholder concept

b) social contract is the key concept of legitimacy theory.

c) Key concept of enlightened self-interest is stakeholder relations.

d) Stakeholder theory require organizations to manage community perceptions to survive.

25) Which of the following is correct related to discounting future liabilities?

a) Discounting future cash flows is not aligned with the aims and objectives of sustainability report.

b) Discounting future costs that are to be incurred increases the current liability.

c) Discounting future costs highlights the savings of the future generations due to present generations accounting.

d) Discounting social issues are done in terms of the accounting standards so that there are no ethical issues.

26) High commitment approach to environmental issues may include all of the following

a) Risk analysis

b) Stakeholder analysis

c) Green washing

d) Strategic sustainability auditing

27) Which of the following statements regarding institutional shareholders is correct?

a) Have extensive power to monitor activities of the company.

b) Prefer to exert their power privately rather than publicly.

c) Aim to improve outcomes rather than sell their shareholding.

d) Institutional shares are known to publicly use their voting power to encourage sound corporate decision-making.

e) Both A and D.

28) Which of the following is not a driver of responsible competitive-ness?

a) Policy drivers

b) Development drivers

c) Business action

d) Social enablers

29 Unbounded solution in an LPP is

a) Where the objective function can be decreased indefinitely.

b) Which maximizes the objective function

c) Where the objective function can be increased or decreased indefinitely.

d) Where the objective function can be increased indefinitely.

30) The objective of the transportation problem is to

a) Maximize the total profit

b) Minimize the total loss

c) Neither maximize nor minimize

d) Optimal cost

31) Which market structure witness a demand kink, as the curve is more elastic above the kink and less elastic below it has because customer response to a price increase is less than the response to a price decrease.

a) Monopoly

b) Monopolistic competition

c) Oligopoly

d) Duopoly

32) Equilibrium is determined at the levels of output were

1. MC=MR

2. MC>MR

3. MC<MR

a) Both 2 and 3

b) Both 1 and 3

c) Both 1 and 3

d) None of the above

33) According to the managerial grid, which of the following management styles can be exercised by the organization.

a) Country club management, b) Team management, c) Improvised management, d) charismatic management

b) Country club management, b) Team management, c) Situational management. d) Task management

c) Country club management, b) Team management c) Impoverished, d) Task Management

34) Is the finite time and time that senior managers in a company possess. It is most often discussed when discussing the role and responsibilities of leaders and that many leaders take on more time than they can cry.

a) Administrative Theory

b) Scientific Management

c) Bandwidth Management

d) Management Bandwidth

e) Systems Management Theory

35) Customer decides not to join the queue by seeing the number of customers already in service system.

a) Balking

b) Reneging

c) Jockeying

d) Patient Customer

36) Customer after joining the queue, waits for some time and leaves the service due to delay in service.

a) Reneging

b) Jockeying

c) Balking

d) Impatient customer

37) If an activity has a total float of 10 minutes, with the latest start at 15th minute, then its earliest start is

a) 25 minutes

b) 10 minutes

c) 5 minutes

d) None of the above

38) If a project activity has pessimistic time of 9 minutes and optimistic time of 1 minute, with its most likely completion in 5 minutes. Then the expected activity duration is

a) 5 minutes

b) 2.56 minutes

c) 3.5 minutes

d) 9 minutes

39) A distribution which has equal tails, with a halving process of entire set of observations is called

a) Binomial distribution

b) Poisson Distribution

c) Beta Distribution

d) Normal Gaussian Distribution

40) A distribution of probability calculated by multiplying the probability of success raised to the power of the number of the successes and the probability of failure raised to the power of the difference between the number of is called

a) Poisson distribution

b) Gamma distribution

c) Cumulative Density Distribution

d) None of the above

41) **Promotion of Zara Hatke Movie is**

a) One to One marketing

b) Door to door selling

c) Road Show

d) Online promotion

e) Informative advertising

42) **If Vicky Kaushal vibes on obsessed personalized only for you, this is called**

a) Inter-personal communication

b) Extrinsic motivation

c) Attitude

d) Intrinsic motivation

e) Personality

43) **According to you, which product is correctly combined with Market structure**

a) Inferior goods- Perfect competition

b) Superior goods- Monopoly

c) Veblen goods - Monopolistic competition

d) Normal goods - oligopoly

44) **Which of the following are modes of GAT's for supply of a service**

a) Cross border

b) Consumption abroad

c) Commercial presence

d) All of the above

e) None of the above

45) **Which of the following is not a vertical of World Bank Group?**

a) IBRD

b) International Development Association (IDA)

c) General Agreement on Trade and Tariffs (GATTS)

d) The International Finance Corporation (IFC)

e) The Multilateral Investment Guarantee Agency (MIGA)

46) **Identify incorrect formula**

a) Sales-FC/EBIT

b) EBIT/EBT= Financial Leverage

c) Contribution - FC/EBIT-Interest = Financial Leverage

d) Contribution - FC/EBIT = Financial Leverage

47) **Which theory states that "Consistency in judgement of people or issues linked by some form of relationship. Relationship of 3 elements- person, other person, impersonal entity, forming 2 relations- sentiment and unit (+ve,-ve)**

a) Balance theory

b) Cognitive dissonance theory

c) Cognitive theory

d) None of the above

e) Alderfer ERG Theory

48) **The following statement is true according to which theory - When cognitive components are incongruent, people will be motivated to alter their attitudes or behaviour to bring the whole back into balance.**

a) Cognitive dissonance theory

b) Maslow's need hierarchy

c) ERG theory of motivation

d) Consistency theory of attitude

49) **Identify the correct combination**

a) MASLOW- ERG

b) PAC- Leadership Style

c) RoE- Accounting Concepts and Convention

d) NOI-Capital structure

e) None of the above

50) Which of the following is not an advantage of strategic management?

a) Provides organizations with a clear sense of direction and purpose.

b) Helps improve the political, economic, social and technological environment of the organization

c) Helps to orientate management decisions to relevant environment conditions

d) None of the above

51) Which of the following is not a characteristic of strategic management that makes it different from other type of management?

a) It is interdisciplinary

b) Has external focus

c) Has internal focus

d) Concerns present direction of the organization

52) The fundamental of an organization's mission statement is to

a) Create a good human relations climate in the organization

b) To define organization's purpose in society

c) Define organizational structure of the organization

d) Generate good public relations for the organization

53) If firm is at BEP, with FC of Rs 3 L and variable cost as 50% of sales. Calculate units sold for selling price @ Rs 150/unit

a) 1500

b) 5000

c) 4000

d) 4900

e) 490

f) 1789

54) Receiving job satisfaction from your company is

a) Satisfier according to Herzberg 2-factor theory

b) Self Realization according to Maslow's need theory

c) Physiological need according to Maslow's need theory

d) None of the above

55) The board of directors' work on behalf of stakeholders, this model is referred to as

a) Stakeholders model

b) Agency model

c) Ethical model

d) Anglo-Saxon model

56) If ABC Ltd issued 20% debentures for Rs. 5 L and 1000 shares for Rs 15 L. EBIT is Rs 2 L Calculate D/E ratio and EAT if tax rate is 40%

a) 3:1, Rs 60,000

b) 2:1, Rs 1,00,000

c) 1:3, Rs 67,000

d) 1:3, Rs 40,000

e) 1:3, Rs 60,000

57) A leader calls in suggestions from his team members to improve customer satisfaction. Such style is called

a) Autocratic

b) Situational

c) Charismatic

d) None of the above

58) ____ is RBI mandated system that offers integrated and interoperable bill payment services to customers across geographies to customers across geographies with certainty, reliability and safety of transactions.

a) UPI

b) Internet Banking

c) Mobile Banking

d) Bharat Bill Payment System

e) All of the above

f) None of the above

59) If an organization cleanliness is not maintained every day, it will lead to extrinsic demotivation, leading to violation of which theory

a) Law of Demand

b) Law of Invariable Proportion

c) Maslow's need theory

d) Alderfer ERG theory

e) Herzberg's 2 factor theory.

60) If firm issues 20 % dividend ratio for earnings per share of Rs 250, what is dividend paid?

a) Rs 25

b) Rs 65

c) Rs 50

d) None of the above

61) Which of the following explains that number of units of one product that can be increased by reducing the quantity of another product?

a) Marginal rate of substitution

b) Marginal rate of propensity

c) Marginal rate of transformation

d) All of the above

62) Which of the following explains that the amount of a good that a consumer is willing to consume as compared to another good, as long as the new good is equally satisfying:

a) Propensity to come

b) Demand function

c) Marginal rate of Substitution

d) Marginal rate of propensity

63) Which of the following is studied to evaluate how much quantity is to be produced by the firm?

a) Demand function

b) Cost function

c) Supply function

d) All of the above

64) Which body is responsible for printing/circulating Commemorative Coins in India

a) SEBI

b) UGC

c) RBI

d) SPMCIL (Security Printing and Minting Corporation of India Limited)

65) Which body is responsible for currency sterilization in India?

a) SEBI

b) Ministry of Corporate Affairs

c) UGC

d) AICTE

e) CABE

f) None of the above

66) If an investor sells below exercise price, on expiration date, then he will

a) Gain

b) Loose

c) No gain no loose

d) None of the above

67) Which ratio is useful if the firm wants to analyse the source of capital weightage?

a) Return on Investments Ratio

b) Return on Equity Ratio

c) Debt-Equity Ratio

d) Current Assets-Current Liabilities Ratio

68) Identify the type of marketing analysis that relies on data and insights to improve ROI, similar to data driven marketing where in sales and marketing teams work together to report on led in endless feedback:

a) Word of mouth marketing

b) Digital marketing

c) Closed loop marketing

d) Both A and B

69) Which of the following can be checked by a potential investor before investing in an organization:

a) Balance sheet

b) Income/P&L statement

c) EBIT-EPS Analysis

d) Net Operating Income

e) Dividend Payout Ratio

70) RBI's clean note policy was introduced in

a) 2019, RBI Governor Dr Ustad Amjad Ali Khan

b) 1999, RBI Governer, Dr. Bimal Jain

c) 2001, RBI Governer, Dr. Nirmala S

d) 2007, RBI Governer, Dr. Radhe Shyam Tiwari

71) OD process is cyclical and ends when

a) Desired development result is obtained.

b) Plan is implemented

c) Data is gathered

d) Problem is identified

72) The organizational diagnosis means-

a) To identify strength and weaknesses problem areas

b) To find out discrepancies, between vision and desired future and current situations

c) Both A and B

d) None of the above

73) OD was founded on the belief that using behavioural sciences methods to increase collaborative problem solving would increase

a) Organizational effectiveness

b) Organizational turnover

c) Organizational reputation

d) All of the above

74) OD Intervention seminars being conducted in the organisations help to

a) Improve overall efficiency

b) Improve productivity

c) Improve morale of employees

d) All the above

75) Which of the following is a performance management technique:

a) Essays

b) Write-ups

c) Observations

d) All of the above

e) None of the above

76) Which of the following is necessary for entrepreneurs to prepare when

applying for venture capital or seeking seed capital from financers.

a) Business Report

b) Annual Financial Report

c) Feasibility analysis and Business Plan

d) None of the above

77) **Which of the following statement is true?**

a) R is equal to +0.80, there is a strong positive correlation in variables

b) R is equal to +0.80, there is a strong negative correlation in variables

c) R is equal to +0.98, there is a weak positive correlation in variables

d) R is equal to (-)0 .15, there is a strong weak correlation in variables

78) **According to which theory, a country is said to have better hand at production and export of a product.**

a) Mercantilism Theory

b) Hecker-Ohlin Theory

c) Absolute Advantage Theory

d) Comparative Advantage Theory

79) **A firm with 2.50 current ratio and current liabilities half of Total Liabilities. What are Current assets, if Total liabilities stand at Rs.15 Lacs.**

a) Rs.45 Lac

b) Rs.37.5 Lac

c) Rs.18.75 Lac

d) Rs.12.85 Lac.

80) **STATEMENT I - Under Organisation development theory, Forming and norming stage of group formulation suggests that group so formed according to the needs will function till the life span of the organisation.**

STATEMENT II - Under simulation training technique, staff undergoes training in a make-shift setup or dummy set-up, which is on the same lines of the real-life scenario of the job.

a. Both STATEMENT I and STATEMENT II are correct.

b. Both STATEMENT I and STATEMENT II are incorrect.

c. STATEMENT I is correct and STATEMENT II is incorrect.

d. STATEMENT I is incorrect and STATEMENT II is correct.

81) **When the investor writes a put option and has no position in the underlying stock then such strategy is called**

a) Covered call

b) Butterfly spread

c) Married Put

d) Bull call spread

e) Naked Put

82) **Most occurring phenomenon in classrooms is**

a) Use of lecture method

b) Use of teaching aids

c) Use of high-tech teaching methods

d) Use of memory level strategies

1) A, B, C

2) B, C, D

3) A, C, D

4) B and D

83) **ANSWER WHETHER THE FOLLOWING STATEMENT(S) ARE CORRECT OR INCORRECT: STATEMENT I: According to the Hofstede Cultural Dimensions theory, firms across countries have same cultural norms**

towards power distance, between the boss and the peers. STATEMENT II: According to the Hofstede Cultural Dimensions theory, the employees avoiding uncertainty the most find themselves to be unexpected situations the most.

a) Both STATEMENT I and STATEMENT II are correct.

b) Both STATEMENT I and STATEMENT II are incorrect.

c) STATEMENT I is correct and STATEMENT II is incorrect.

d) STATEMENT I is incorrect and STATEMENT II is correct.

84) ANSWER WHETHER THE FOLLOWING STATEMENT(S) ARE CORRECT OR INCORRECT: STATEMENT I: According to the Hofstede Cultural Dimensions theory, a firm with more role differentiation due to gender is stuck in traditional system of masculinity and feminism. STATEMENT II: According to the Hofstede Cultural Dimensions theory, the employees with short-term orientation attain short-term success.

a) Both STATEMENT I and STATEMENT II are correct.

b) Both STATEMENT I and STATEMENT II are incorrect.

c) STATEMENT I is correct and STATEMENT II is incorrect.

d) STATEMENT I is incorrect and STATEMENT II is correct.

85) ANSWER WHETHER THE FOLLOWING STATEMENT(S) ARE CORRECT OR INCORRECT: STATEMENT I: According to the Trait theory, leaders are borne with leadership qualities such as confidence, intelligence, etc. STATEMENT II: According to the Situational leadership theory, leaders keep on changing their respective style of leadership according to the situation.

a) Both STATEMENT I and STATEMENT II are correct.

b) Both STATEMENT I and STATEMENT II are incorrect.

c) STATEMENT I is correct and STATEMENT II is incorrect.

d) STATEMENT I is incorrect and STATEMENT II is correct.

86) ANSWER WHETHER THE FOLLOWING STATEMENT(S) ARE CORRECT OR INCORRECT: STATEMENT I: According to the Four temperaments theory, a choleric personality has a changeable disposition. STATEMENT II: According to the Four temperaments theory, a sanguine personality is calm and persistent.

a) Both STATEMENT I and STATEMENT II are correct.

b) Both STATEMENT I and STATEMENT II are incorrect.

c) STATEMENT I is correct and STATEMENT II is incorrect.

d) STATEMENT I is incorrect and STATEMENT II is correct.

87) ANSWER WHETHER THE FOLLOWING STATEMENT(S) ARE CORRECT OR INCORRECT: STATEMENT I: According to the functions of attitude, an individual who protects his self-image and avoids threats has the self-expressive function. STATEMENT II: In the theory of reasoned action, consumer intention to perform the act of purchasing is always attached with a reason to purchase.

a) Both STATEMENT I and STATEMENT II are correct.

b) Both STATEMENT I and STATEMENT II are incorrect.

c) STATEMENT I is correct and STATEMENT II is incorrect.

d) STATEMENT I is incorrect and STATEMENT II is correct.

88) **ANSWER WHETHER THE FOLLOWING STATEMENT(S) ARE CORRECT OR INCORRECT: STATEMENT I: According to the cognitive dissonance theory, people who are motivated to purchase have more of inconsistent buying behaviour. STATEMENT II: In the Multi-attribute model, a consumer associates same likeness towards a product, with every brand he evaluates before the purchasing decision.**

a) Both STATEMENT I and STATEMENT II are correct.

b) Both STATEMENT I and STATEMENT II are incorrect.

c) STATEMENT I is correct and STATEMENT II is incorrect.

d) STATEMENT I is incorrect and STATEMENT II is correct.

89) **ANSWER WHETHER THE FOLLOWING STATEMENT(S) ARE CORRECT OR INCORRECT: STATEMENT I: According to the Kantianism theory of business ethics, consequences are disregarded. STATEMENT II: In the Stakeholders theory, firm management has responsibility towards all its stakeholders.**

a) Both STATEMENT I and STATEMENT II are correct.

b) Both STATEMENT I and STATEMENT II are incorrect.

c) STATEMENT I is correct and STATEMENT II is incorrect.

d) STATEMENT I is incorrect and STATEMENT II is correct.

90) **ANSWER WHETHER THE FOLLOWING STATEMENT(S) ARE CORRECT OR INCORRECT-STATEMENT I: White papers do not involve extensive researches. STATEMENT II: White papers are another name for research papers, there is no difference in both.**

a) Both STATEMENT I and STATEMENT II are correct.

b) Both STATEMENT I and STATEMENT II are incorrect.

c) STATEMENT I is correct and STATEMENT II is incorrect.

d) STATEMENT I is incorrect and STATEMENT II is correct.

91) **ANSWER WHETHER THE FOLLOWING STATEMENT(S) ARE CORRECT OR INCORRECT-STATEMENT I: Understanding research process helps researchers to reduce biases from research. STATEMENT II: Biases and ethical practices occur simultaneously.**

a) Both STATEMENT I and STATEMENT II are correct.

b) Both STATEMENT I and STATEMENT II are incorrect.

c) STATEMENT I is correct and STATEMENT II is incorrect.

d) STATEMENT I is incorrect and STATEMENT II is correct.

92) **ANSWER WHETHER THE FOLLOWING STATEMENT(S) ARE CORRECT OR INCORRECT-STATEMENT I: Use of unethical means can be hided in research reports, by researchers. STATEMENT II: Research report format APA is used for science-field driven researches.**

a) Both STATEMENT I and STATEMENT II are correct.

b) Both STATEMENT I and STATEMENT II are incorrect.

c) STATEMENT I is correct and STATEMENT II is incorrect.

d) STATEMENT I is incorrect and STATEMENT II is correct.

93) **ANSWER WHETHER THE FOLLOWING STATEMENT(S) ARE CORRECT OR INCORRECT-STATEMENT I: Plagiarism occurs when a researcher presents and publishes his research in a university Seminar and journal. STATEMENT II: Mosaic plagiarism is to use ones 'own research at another seminar.**

a) Both STATEMENT I and STATEMENT II are correct.

b) Both STATEMENT I and STATEMENT II are incorrect.

c) STATEMENT I is correct and STATEMENT II is incorrect.

d) STATEMENT I is incorrect and STATEMENT II is correct.

94) **ANSWER WHETHER THE FOLLOWING STATEMENT(S) ARE CORRECT OR INCORRECT-STATEMENT I: Use of data collection tools can help prepare a carefully well-planned research proposal. STATEMENT II: Use of hypothesis tests on qualitative data, such as Z-, F-, T- gives necessary data insights.**

a) Both STATEMENT I and STATEMENT II are correct.

b) Both STATEMENT I and STATEMENT II are incorrect.

c) STATEMENT I is correct and STATEMENT II is incorrect.

d) STATEMENT I is incorrect and STATEMENT II is correct.

95) **ANSWER WHETHER THE FOLLOWING STATEMENT(S) ARE CORRECT OR INCORRECT-STATEMENT I: Self plagiarism occurs when one uses too many references, citations in research report. STATEMENT II: Hidden responses can seeked by researchers, by using disguised observation techniques.**

a) Both STATEMENT I and STATEMENT II are correct.

b) Both STATEMENT I and STATEMENT II are incorrect.

c) STATEMENT I is correct and STATEMENT II is incorrect.

d) STATEMENT I is incorrect and STATEMENT II is correct.

96) **ANSWER WHETHER THE FOLLOWING STATEMENT(S) ARE CORRECT OR INCORRECT-STATEMENT I: Mostly researchers tend not to obtain informed consent from respondents. STATEMENT II: Not giving citations is a severe case of plagiarism and ethical practices, done by researchers.**

a) Both STATEMENT I and STATEMENT II are correct.

b) Both STATEMENT I and STATEMENT II are incorrect.

c) STATEMENT I is correct and STATEMENT II is incorrect.

d) STATEMENT I is incorrect and STATEMENT II is correct.

97) **ANSWER WHETHER THE FOLLOWING STATEMENT(S) ARE CORRECT OR INCORRECT-Statement I: Qualitative research seeks out the 'why', not the 'how' of its topic through the analysis of unstructured information - things like interview transcripts, e-mails, notes, feedback forms, photos and videos.** Statement II:-

Quantitative research is used to help us understand how people feel and why they feel as they do. It is concerned with collecting in-depth information asking questions such as why do you say that? Choose the correct options from below:

a) Both Statement I and Statement II are correct.

b) Both Statement I and Statement II are incorrect.

c) Statement I is correct but Statement II is incorrect.

d) Statement I is incorrect but Statement II is correct.

98) **ANSWER WHETHER THE FOLLOWING STATEMENT(S) ARE CORRECT OR INCORRECT-STATEMENT I: Secondary data is information gathered for purposes other than the completion of a research project. STATEMENT II: A variety of secondary information sources is available to the researcher gathering data on an industry, potential product applications and the market place. Secondary data is also used to gain initial insight into the research problem. Choose the correct options from below:**

a) Both Statement I and Statement II are correct.

b) Both Statement I and Statement II are incorrect.

c) Statement I is correct but Statement II is incorrect.

d) Statement I is incorrect but Statement II is correct.

99) **ANSWER WHETHER THE FOLLOWING STATEMENT(S) ARE CORRECT OR INCORRECT-STATEMENT I: The quickest and the cheapest way to formulate a hypothesis in research is by using Literature Search. STATEMENT II: When secondary data is available, the researcher need only locate the source of the data and extract the required information. Choose the correct options from below:**

a) Both Statement I and Statement II are correct.

b) Both Statement I and Statement II are incorrect.

c) Statement I is correct but Statement II is incorrect.

d) Statement I is incorrect but Statement II is correct.

100) **ANSWER WHETHER THE FOLLOWING STATEMENT(S) ARE CORRECT OR INCORRECT-STATEMENT I: In Descriptive Research Design it is essentially a research to describe Quantitative data. STATEMENT II: Descriptive study requires a clear specification of "Who, what, when, where, why and how" of the research. Choose the correct options from below:**

a) Both Statement I and Statement II are correct.

b) Both Statement I and Statement II are incorrect.

c) Statement I is correct but Statement II is incorrect.

d) Statement I is incorrect but Statement II is correct.

Answer Key Mock Test - 7

1) C: The concept of time value of money suggests that over the time. Rates of interest help consumers appreciate their investment in terms of countering the prevailing inflation rates it is often seen that interest rates are a little more than the prevailing inflation rates suggesting that over the time Money appreciates, hence Giving the impression that there is a value of time involved in appreciating money as investment.
2) B: Gaining consumers by advertising at low prices, with no intention to sell it but persuading customer to buy a costlier version.
3) B:. Career management is defined as an activity initiated by the hour of an employee who get involved to help him manage his career and enhance his resume with the help of various skills related to his career and existing work.
4) B: Bread crumbling follows the principle of intermittent relationship, which is a psychological concept. It can create a mixture of feelings of hope and disappointment, Keeping the employee engaged with no or very little work.
5) C: Mom and pop store also called as Kiryana store are local groceries and general store located in the vicinity of a residential society these stores offer very less variety and house very less number of units of various products the mom and pop store believe in keeping most essential daily usage items in Max quantity.
6) D: It is often seen that a low engagement from the bosses or the organization results in the situation of an employee taking a unhappy leave in which he feels disengaged towards his job and would like to take a break for a short duration.
7) A: The maternity benefits act is specifically designed to help working women cope up with their maternity with the help of monetary and non-monetary benefits extended by their employers.
8) C: The marketing concept for an organization is the guiding light to help them device a marketing and an advertising strategy for the near and distant future.
9) B: Online apps which take and receive orders for customers open up dark stores in order to make sure that the products and the customer orders are dispersed these dark stores are not used for direct contact with consumers for retaining purpose.
10) A: Stagflation is a type of inflation wherein the inflation exists in the market and in food prices, etc. but the inflation rate remains stagnant and does not change a lot. Since the mean height is a huge two-digit number, it is suggestive that the population is large from which the sample is drawn.
11) C: For a country which operates on the economics of discrimination makes sure that the economic cycle keeps on going by not providing employment to the entire countryman and making sure that few of the citizens are entangled in qualification, some are entangled in selection processes and the rest are working as employed personnels.
12) B: Depending on the inflation rates an increase in income does not warranty that every time expenditure will tend to increase if there is any increase in income it might suggest that the employee might end up increasing their savings or might be increasing their expenditure depending on the inflation rates prevailing in the country at that point of time.

13) B: Explanation- NA
14) B: Due to the fact that the firm in moving towards stability stage of its product and firm life cycle, it will be bought at a less rate and sold at higher rate, to make profits.
15) B: Using the 360 degree performance appraisal technique the HR for an employee is able to gather qualitative quantitative assessment report from his various subordinates peers and superiors.
16) D: The hertzberg two factor theory is focused on two factors which help in employees stay motivated to work in an organization including hygiene factors and job based recognition.
17) D: In order to help organizations save on their taxes they enter into certain arrangements with their employees wherein they pay a higher salary only to take back certain portion of it in cash showing as total salary of expenses and thereof helping organization reduce its tax liabilities.
18) A: This doctrine suggests that no law is going to hold true forever and as the changing economics suggest for a country any law or provision might undergo severability depending on its application on the citizens time to time.
19) C: Explanation- NA
20) C: Harmonious relationships between managers and subordinates help the dynamics of the organization to be implemented smoothly managers who work with subordinates and bosses need to make sure that external parties such as suppliers stakeholders consumers are all satisfied with the workings and operations of the organisation over the time. To help organisation keep on running smoothly.
21) B: Under section 45ZB, of the RBI Act, 1934, a statutory body has to be formulated within RBI, whose principle role is to look into the inflation rate changes and formulate/recommend monetary policy changes to combat inflation to the Monetary policy committee.
22) A: Ceremonial duties of a manager include motivational meetings pep up talks with their subordinates 1 to 1 rounds of performance review this helps them build a professional relationship with their subordinates. Any kind of communication which flows in the organization as top-down or bottom-up approach helps the managers keep informed themselves in order to let the work happen smoothly.
23) A: Every function within the organization is assigned with the managerial position in order to make sure that the work of that functional area is smoothly implemented for example for human resource function there is a hour manager for accounting function there is an accounts manager in an organization where the production needs to be supervised the product or the service both get supervised in terms of manufacturing and delivering it thereof.
24) B: Foreign organization to practice their CSR responsibilities they need to understand the business will be legitimate only when they are able to disperse CSR basis for the benefit of the society at large from whom they are sharing the resources time and again.
25) A: The sustainability report is a qualitative analysis of the organization to help the stakeholders understand how the organization plans to manage its longevity in the dynamics of the prevailing economic conditions. Whereas the concept of discounting future cash inflows and outflows rests upon the principle of time value of money which helps us calculate the net present value of distant cash flows.

26) C: The concept of greenwashing is entered into by an organization who wishes to keep the customers and stakeholders under dark by manipulating their figures and doing the act of grain washing through means of their annual report and financial statements.

27) E: Institutional investors are routine nature investors who give lend money to the organization and keep on monitoring the implementation of cash flows within the organization and during stress times for the business cycle do not for sale their shareholding rather encourage organizations to improvise their operations.

28) B: Development drivers DO NOT contribute towards market competitiveness; they exist at company level and hence are individual to each firm/ sector/country.

29) C: Since the solution in the Linear programming problem is falling outside the area on bounded solution (graphically), the unbounded region in the graph has scope of expansion, thereby leading to scope of the objective function to increase or decrease according to the problem verticals, indefinitely.

30) A: Transportation problems help calculate total and optimal costs to be incurred according to the initial feasible solution or the MODI Method of optimization leading to least cost being found and thereby maximizing on the profits.

31) B: Under monopolistic competition, demand related kinks are witnessed in the demand curve, wherein the price decrease by the firms lead to increase in demand adding to the elasticity function and an increase in price is not causing immediate major impact, therefore leading to a slight rigidity in increase in consumption, later adding to less of elasticity.

32) B: If the marginal revenue is equal to marginal cost, so that the costs incurred are being recovered from the goods sold, the firm keeps going with the existing rate of production, and when the revenue is greater than the marginal costs incurred, the firm plans to increase the rate of production from the current levels.

33) D: Explanation- NA

34) D: Explanation- NA

35) A: Explanation- NA

36) A: Explanation- NA

37) C: Earliest start is when the activity can begin, latest start is the maximum time it might take to begin, total float is the duration taken by the activity being performed.

38) A: Mean = [O+4M+P]/6 = [30]/6 = 5 Minutes.

39) D: Halving process involves data being reduced by a factor 2 in order to truncate or bring it to half-normal distribution.

40) D: A distribution of probability calculated by multiplying the probability of success raised to the power of the number of the successes and the probability of failure raised to the power of the difference between the number of is called as binomial distribution.

41) E: Any promotion which give details about the product/service is called as informative advertising.

42) B: Extrinsic motivation is a source which lies outside the individual and such motivation comes from the external environment of the individual.

43) C: In a perfect competitive market, goods are homogenous due to normal profits to the firm and many firms offering same product type. In monopolistic competition, the Veblen goods are a degree better than normal but a degree less than superior products.

44) D: The GATS distinguishes between four modes of supplying services: cross-border trade, consumption abroad, commercial presence, and presence of natural persons.

45) C: World bank is a group of 5 verticals- International Bank for Reconstruction and Development-
- International Development Association.
- International Finance Corporation.
- Multilateral Investment Guarantee Agency.
- International Centre for Settlement of Investment Disputes.

46) A: Correct Formula = [Sales-Variable Cost]/EBIT

47) A: Balance theory suggests that the groups when formed with individuals who have same value system, beliefs, attitudes.

48) A: When an individual is not able to process the inputs and stimulus he receives from his environment(internal/ external) Is said to be dissonant cognitively.

49) D: Capital Structure theories include - Net operating income approach, Net income approach, suggesting that the firm value depends on its operational sales and the other suggesting that the less of debt component the greater will be the value of firm, as available for distribution to shareholders.

50) D: Explanation- NA

51) D: Strategic management is a future oriented aspect of the firm. It does guide the present scenario only to better improve the future of the firm.

52) B: A firm prepares a Vision (Philosophical statement about the existence of the firm) and a Mission statement (clearly citing the reason for its existence in a more precise manner, with more emphasis on stakeholders).

53) C: [Sales-Variable Cost] = Contribution - Fixed Cost = Profit/Loss/BEP.[x-50% of x] = 3 Lac - 3 Lac = NIL (BEP). VC = 50% of Sales and hence Contribution = 50%6 Lac - 3 Lac = 3 Lac (Sales - VC = Contribution).Sales in units = 6 Lac/ 150 per unit = 4000 units.

54) A: According to the Herzberg 2-factor theory, a firm can extrinsically motivate employees through Hygiene factors and Motivation factors (Recognition/ enrichment).

55) B: The firm directors are agents of the stakeholder and need to run and manage the company on behalf of the stakeholders, as their agents.

56) E: EBIT - Interest = EBT - Tax = EAT.2 Lac - (20% of 5 Lac) = 1 Lac - 40000 = 60,000.D/E = 500,000/15,00,000 = 1.3.

57) D: Since this is not a particular situation to ask suggests and the leader is not leading through charisma.

58) D: Explanation- NA

59) E: According to the Herzberg 2-factor theory, a firm can extrinsically motivate employees through Hygiene factors and Motivation factors (Recognition/ enrichment).

60) C: Dividend Payout Ratio (DPR) = Dividend per share / Earnings per share.0.20 = x / 250 X = 0.20 * 250 = Rs.50

61) C: For a new product launched as a variant, the firm can opt to bundle both the products if their features are only slightly similar or launch it with minor reduction in availability of parent product.

62) C: Substitution effects take place when a product is temporarily unavailable and the firm is slightly replacing it with new goods.

63) C: Supply function determines the supplier/manufacturer side input to the market in terms of finished goods.

64) D: Explanation- NA

65) F: In a country, currency sterilization practice is undertaken by the central bank of the country, in order to impact

the foreign exchange rates of the currency and to stabilize the money supply of the home currency.

66) B: Selling on expiration date is NOT shorting the position, but the sale happens to be below the exercise price, suggests that the option is out of money and has not generated profits for the holder.

67) C: Debt-equity ratio will help firm understand the weights the two sources have on the total capital raise by the firm.

68) C: Both marketing and sales team analyze the consumer driven data to develop future strategies to optimize on advertising and marketing.

69) C: EBIT-EPS Analysis helps understand the earnings potential of the firm and various expenses it incurs and the earnings which shareholders earn per share.

70) B.

71) A: The process of organizational development is an ongoing and never ending process due to the ever changing dynamics of the environment in which the firm operates.

72) C: Through environmental scanning an organization can understand about Strength and weakness through internal analysis and align them according to the available opportunities and threat pertinent in the external environment.

73) A: Organizational effectiveness is when the firm is able to produce results, using any and all macro & micro factors to better itself even during stress times in the business environment.

74) D: Intervention seminars are towards organization development, for improving employee performance and firm efficiency.

75) C: Observations help managers understand the employees better, specifically when they are on the job and actively engaged.

76) C: Feasibility analysis refers to a set of documents supporting the business plan in terms of marketing, operations, financing, etc and Business Plan is document carrying all necessary information of the business/business model, etc.

77) A: The correlation value of two variable responses ranges between 0.01 to 1.00 is a positive correlation else if the correlation falls between -0.01 to -1.0, the correlation is said to have negative association between the variables. If the correlation ranges between 0.50 to 1.0 is said to be strongly positive correlation of the given variables.

78) D: The comparative advantage theory suggests that among the given two countries A and B, one country is said to have advantage over the other in terms of available factor of production (Raw material/labour/Capital).

79) C: Current Liabilities is half of Total Liabilities (Rs.15 Lac) = Rs.7.5 Lac.Current Ratio = Current Assets/ Current Liabilities2.5 = x/7.5 Lac X = 7.5 Lac * 2.5 = Rs.18.75 Lac.

80) D: Under Organisation development theory, Forming and norming stage of group formulation suggests that group so formed according to the needs, will function till the objective of the group formed is to be met.

81) E

82) 3) A, C, D

83) B: According to the Hofstede Cultural Dimensions theory, firms across countries have different cultural dimensions, such as the power distance index shared between the boss and the peers.According to the Hofstede Cultural Dimensions theory, the employees with high uncertainty avoidance have less tolerance towards ambiguity and prefer high involvement of rules in their lives.

84) A: According to the Hofstede Cultural Dimensions theory, a firm with more role differentiation due to gender is stuck in traditional and old values system of masculinity and feminism. STATEMENT II: According to the Hofstede Cultural Dimensions theory, the employees with short-term orientation attain short-term success and do not show qualities of endurance.

85) D: According to the Trait theory, leaders are not borne but are made through leadership qualities such as confidence, intelligence, etc. According to the Situational leadership theory, leaders keep on changing their respective style of leadership according to the contingent situation at hand.

86) C: According to the Four temperaments theory, a choleric personality has a changeable disposition, as they change quickly and are hot-headed.According to the Four temperaments theory, a sanguine personality is carefree and easy-going.According to the Four temperaments theory, a phlegmatic personality is calm and persistent.

87) D: According to the functions of attitude, an individual who protects his self-image and avoids threats has the ego-defensive function.In the theory of reasoned action, consumer intention to perform the act of purchasing is always attached with a reason to purchase, such as need of the product, etc.

88) B: According to the cognitive dissonance theory, people who are motivated to purchase often feel the need to separate their buying behaviour pattern from their attitude behind the product being purchased.In the multi-attribute model, a consumer associates different product features, with every brand he evaluates before the purchasing decision.

89) A: According to the Kantianism theory of business ethics, consequences are disregarded but moral duties and rules, regulations are given due importance.In the Stakeholders theory, firm management has responsibility towards all its stakeholders, who might get affected due to the business decisions, being taken at firm level.

90) B: White papers are extensive researches carried on in industrial and practical scenario. And they are different from academically conducted researches called as research papers.

91) C: Understanding of the basic research process helps the researchers prepare for all stages of research step by step, in order to reduces errors, biases to remain ethical in their researches.

92) C: Any unethical and unfair means used in the researches are done with careful precision and are thus hided by the researchers, only to be understood by the very eminent scholars of the field but missed on by the general people. The American psychological association format (APA) is used in business researches, whereas CSE format of research presentation is used for science-driven researches.

93) B: Plagiarism is of various kinds such as mosaic, accidental, etc. mere presentation and publishing of researches is not plagiarism. Plagiarism is faking data/facts/results or copying it from someone else's work. Mosaic plagiarism is using the research work of many other researchers in patches in your own research, without reference citations and is considered unethical manner.

94) C: Mentioning and using data collection methods and tools help prepare every research related document. Hypothesis tests are performed on quantitative data and not qualitative data, since many tests are formula driven.

95) D: Use of many or less references and giving them citations is not a case of self-plagiarism or any other plagiarism since the references are being given to such researches which have been read and considered while conducting own research.In such researches where the respondents get conscious while responding and the research is at the exposure of being comprised due to such responses, therein the researcher with full explanations in his report opt for a disguised method of observation of respondents and collect responses in the truest manner, for example social science driven researches.

96) B: In research methodology, it is always ethical to inform the respondent about the research in general and about any kind of exposures involved and thereafter once the respondents agree the informed consent can be obtained. Which is unlike in case of disguised method of observation. Referring to other research work(s) and not giving reference citation is a case of mosaic plagiarism and is considered to be unethical practice as is termed as copying the work of others.

97) C: Quantitative researches do not work directly on feelings of the respondents unless until they are quantifiable.

98) A: Secondary data can be gathered at the current and used at later stage in career of a researcher in any other research as well, according to the need of the research work.

99) A: Review of literature helps the researcher understand his area of interest and further help him formulate research hypothesis. For any data type, quoting data source is a necessary step in research work, in order to remain ethical throughout.

100) D: Descriptive researches are about qualitative data descriptions or if quantitative data is at first converted to qualitative state and thereafter described about.